QUICK PREP PALEO

50 Fast and Easy Paleo Recipes

MELISSA TAYLOR

TABLE OF CONTENTS

---- BREAKFAST ----

---- LUNCH ----

---- DINNER ----

---- DESSERTS ----

---- SNACKS ----

Breakfast

KALE APPLE SMOOTHIE

Kale is a superfood that you definitely want to be incorporating into your diet.

MAKES 1 SERVING/ TOTAL TIME 10 MINUTE

INGREDIENTS

3/4 cup Kale (chopped, stems removed)

1 Stalk celery (chopped)

1/2 Banana

1/2 cup Apple juice

1/2 cup Ice

1 tablespoon Fresh lemon juice

METHOD

STEP 1
Combine all ingredients in a blender and pulse until smooth.

NUTRITION VALUE	37 Cal, 0.3g fat, 0.05g saturated fat, 1g fiber, 1g protein, 8g carbs.

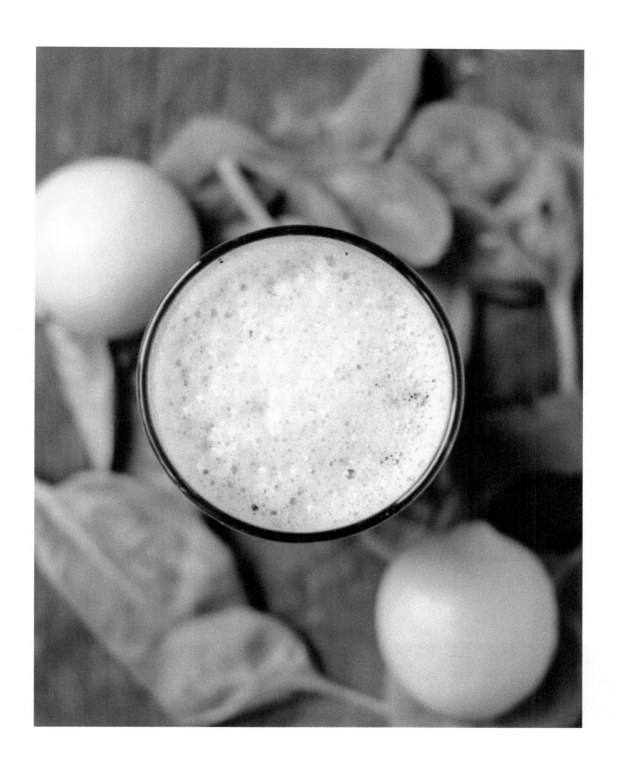

SWEET POTATO BREAKFAST SKILLET

Skillets make for a quick, easy, hearty, and filling breakfast.

MAKES 2 SERVING/ TOTAL TIME 15 MINUTE

INGREDIENTS

1 Onion (large, diced)

3 tbsp Extra virgin olive oil (divided)

2 Italian sausages (diced)

2 Sweet potatoes (finely chopped)

6-7 Stalks asparagus (chopped)

Salt and freshly ground pepper (to taste)

3 Eggs

1 tbsp Fresh parsley (chopped)

METHOD

STEP 1

Heat one tablespoon of olive oil in a large skillet over medium-low heat. Add the onion, sprinkle with salt, and sauté for 10-12 minutes to slightly caramelize.

Add the sausages to the pan and cook for 4-5 minutes. Stir in the sweet potatoes and asparagus, along with another tablespoon of olive oil. Sprinkle with salt and pepper. Cook, covered, for 5-6 minutes, until the potatoes begin to soften. Stir occasionally.

STEP 2

Make three small wells in the sweet potato mixture. Carefully crack the eggs into the wells and cover the skillet. Cook for an additional 5 minutes or until the egg whites are set. Serve immediately, topped with fresh parsley for garnish.

NUTRITION VALUE

199 Cal, 19g fat, 3g saturated fat, 13.6g fiber, 24g protein, 14g carbs.

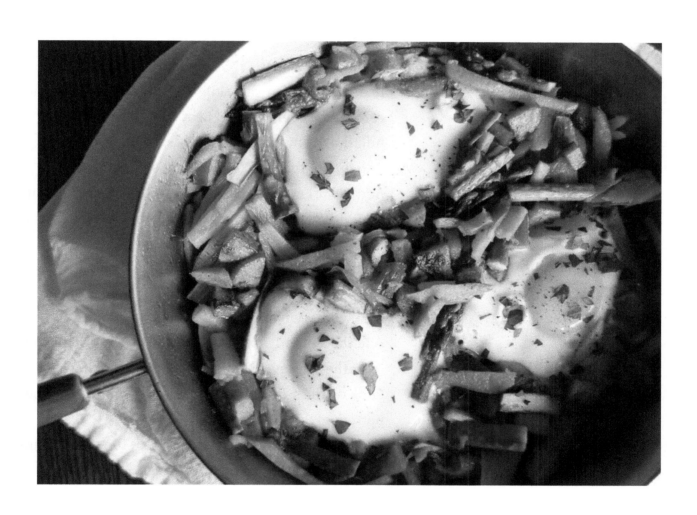

HAM AND BROCCOLI FRITTATA

Frittatas make for delicious, easy breakfasts, and they are also suitable for lunch or even dinner.

MAKES 4 SERVING/ TOTAL TIME 10 MINUTE

INGREDIENTS

8 Eggs

1 tbsp Coconut oil

1/2 Red onion (small, diced)

1 clove garlic (minced)

1/2 Head of broccoli (cut into small florets

1 Sweet potato (small, peeled and finely diced)

1 cup Cooked ham (diced)

1/3 cup Almond milk

1 tbsp Fresh parsley (chopped)

Salt and pepper (to taste)

METHOD

STEP 1

Preheat the oven to 375 degrees F.

In a 10-inch oven-safe skillet or baking dish, melt the coconut oil over medium heat.

Add the onion and sauté for 4-5 minutes until soft.

Add in the garlic and sauté for one minute more.

Add the broccoli into the skillet and cook for 5 minutes.

Add the sweet potato, stirring to combine, and cook for 3-4 minutes.

Stir in the ham.

STEP 2

Meanwhile, whisk the eggs in a medium bowl.

Add the almond milk and season with salt and pepper.

Pour the eggs over the skillet mixture, stirring once.

Cook on the stovetop for 2-3 minutes more to set the bottom of the frittata.

Transfer to the oven and bake for 15-20 minutes, until the eggs are set and cooked through.

NUTRITION VALUE

101 Cal, 6g fat, 4g saturated fat, 1g fiber, 21g protein, 3g carbs.

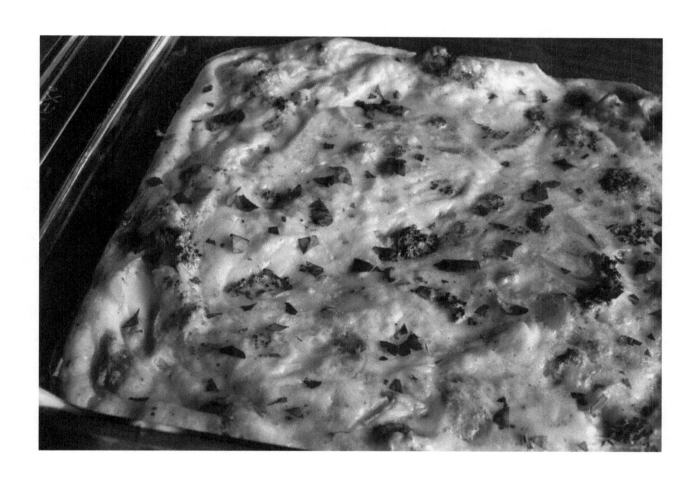

EGGS BENEDICT WITH MUSHROOM HOLLANDAISE

Eggs Benedict makes for a delicious breakfast, though the recipe takes a little extra effort.

MAKES 2 SERVING/ TOTAL TIME 20 MINUTE

INGREDIENTS

1 tsp Extra virgin olive oil

1 Shallot (minced)

2 cups White mushrooms (sliced)

4 Eggs

1 tbsp Apple cider vinegar (for poaching)

Salt and freshly ground pepper (to taste)

Pinch of cayenne

For the sauce

4 Egg yolks

1/4 cup Extra virgin olive oil

3 tbsp Hot water

2 tbsp Lemon juice

Pinch of salt

METHOD

STEP 1

Heat the olive oil in a skillet over medium heat. Add the shallot and sauté for 3-4 minutes. Add the mushrooms and cook for an additional 5 minutes. Transfer the mixture to a bowl and set aside. To poach the eggs, fill the skillet with water and add apple cider vinegar. Heat to barely a simmer. Crack one egg into a small bowl and use the bowl to slowly slide the egg into the water. Cook for 3-4 minutes or until the whites are set and eggs reach preferred level of doneness. Use a slotted spoon to transfer the eggs to a paper towel-lined plate. Repeat with remaining eggs.

STEP 2

For the hollandaise sauce, whisk the egg yolks in a medium metal bowl. Add in the remaining ingredients and continue whisking. Place the bowl over a double-boiler to warm. Whisk constantly until the sauce thickens . Add the mushroom mixture into the bowl and stir to coat. To assemble, divide the poached eggs between two plates.

NUTRITION VALUE	344 Cal, 20g fat, 4g saturated fat, 3g fiber, 21g protein, 10g carbs.

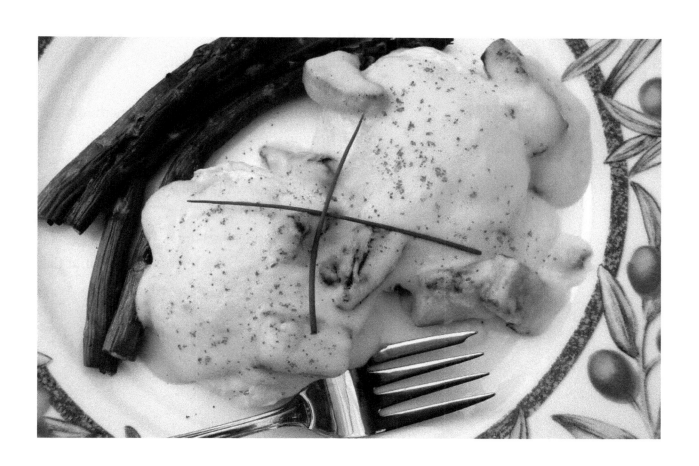

SIMPLE MONKEY SALAD

With its unusual combination of ingredients, the Simple Monkey Salad is both seriously tasty and ridiculously simple. It's a winner!

MAKES 1 SERVING/ TOTAL TIME 10 MINUTE

INGREDIENTS

1 Banana (sliced)

1.5 tbsp Unsweetened coconut flakes

1.5 tbsp Almonds (slivered)

1 tbsp Butter

Drizzle of honey

METHOD

STEP 1

Melt the butter in a small skillet.

Add coconut flakes and almonds.

Toast coconut flakes and almonds on medium heat until golden brown.

STEP 2

Turn off skillet and, while still warm, add drizzle of honey. Mix well.

Slice banana and place in a bowl.

Top banana with toasted almonds and coconut flakes.

Enjoy!

NUTRITION VALUE

234 Cal, 20g fat, 8g saturated fat, 3g fiber, 21g protein, 4g carbs.

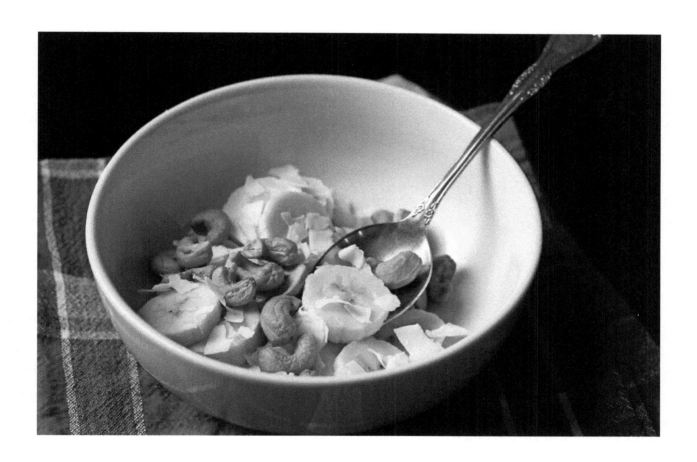

PALEO GRANOLA

This granola is perfect for breakfast, as well as for other meal such as apple crisps .

MAKES 6 SERVING/ TOTAL TIME 30 MINUTE

INGREDIENTS

1/2 c Coconut oil (melted (plus extra for baking sheet))

3/4 c Pumpkin puree

2 tbsp Cinnamon

1/2 tsp Nutmeg

1/4 tsp Cloves

1/4 tsp Allspice

1 tsp Ginger

2 tbsp Vanilla

1 tsp Sea salt

2/3 c Almonds (diced)

1/8 c Chia seeds

2/3 c Pumpkin seeds (pepitas)

3/4 c Unsweetened coconut (shredded)

1 1/2 c Pecans (roughly chopped)

METHOD

STEP 1

Preheat oven to 350 degrees and grease baking sheet with coconut oil. Now is not the time to be stingy. Make it count so that you don't have to scrub that bad boy later!

In a bowl, whisk coconut oil, pumpkin puree, cinnamon, nutmeg, cloves, allspice, ginger, vanilla, and salt. Mix well so that the pumpkin coats the nuts and seeds evenly.

STEP 2

Pour granola mixture onto the baking sheet, and spread out evenly using a spatula.

Bake for about 15-20 minutes, remove the baking sheet, and flip the granola over. Repack evenly using a spatula.

Bake for another 15-20 minutes or until crisp.

Serve with coconut milk, almond milk, or other paleo approved "milk", and enjoy!

NUTRITION VALUE	663 Cal, 20g fat, 12g saturated fat, 1g fiber, 61g protein, 1g carbs.

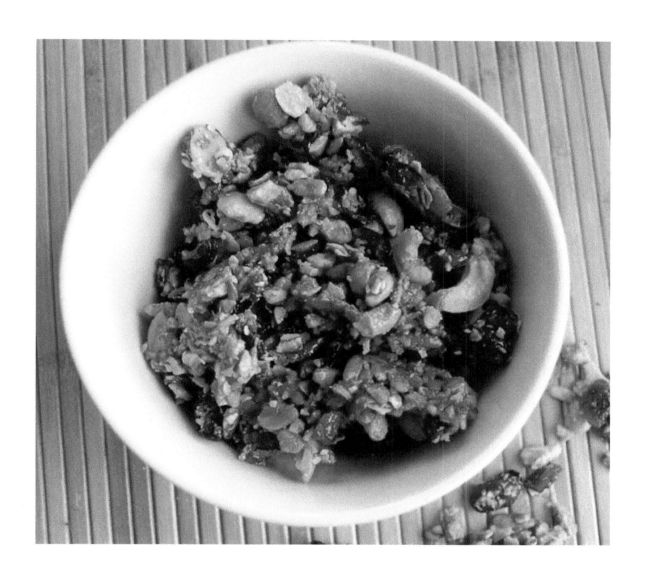

Lunch

CHOCOLATE CHILI STUFFED SWEET POTATO

Sweet potatoes are delicious enough but when you add chocolate chili, your taste buds go crazy.

MAKES 4 SERVING/ TOTAL TIME 20 MINUTE

INGREDIENTS

1 batch Chocolate Chili*

4 Sweet potatoes

METHOD

STEP 1

Preheat oven to 350 degrees and pierce sweet potatoes with a fork.

Pour a tsp or so of olive oil into your hands and grease up each of the sweet potatoes.

STEP 2

Sprinkle potatoes with sea salt and bake for one hour or until they start to drip "sweetness".

Remove sweet potatoes from oven and allow to cool slightly.

Cut open sweet potatoes and top with a generous amount of Chocolate Chili.

Garnish with fresh cut spring onions or chives.

NUTRITION VALUE

646 Cal, 20g fat, 14g saturated fat, 4g fiber, 46g protein, 11g carbs.

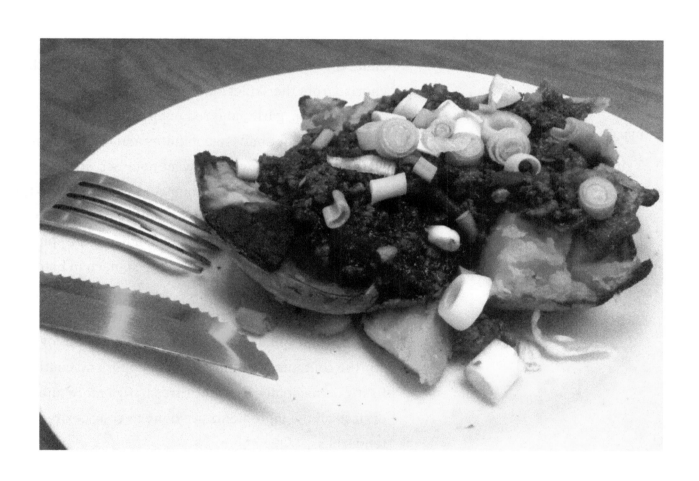

SWEET POTATO HASH WITH CHORIZO

Chorizo is a seasoned sausage that's common in Mexican and Spanish cuisine.

MAKES 2 SERVING/ TOTAL TIME 30 MINUTE

INGREDIENTS

1 Chorizo sausage (Nitrate- and gluten-free, sliced into rounds)

2 cups Baby spinach

1 Sweet potato (peeled and cubed)

2 tbsp Grass fed butter

1/2 cup Red onion (chopped)

2 cloves garlic (minced)

1/4 tsp Red pepper flakes

1/2 tsp Salt

1/2 tsp Black pepper

METHOD

STEP 1

Melt the butter over medium heat in a large skillet. Sauté the chorizo for four to five minutes. Remove the chorizo from the skillet and set aside.

Add the onion, garlic, and red pepper flakes to the skillet. Sauté for about two minutes and then add the sweet potatoes. Brown the sweet potatoes, stirring frequently until just about done. Add the spinach to the skillet with the sweet potatoes. Continue stirring until the sweet potatoes are cooked through and the spinach has wilted. You may have to add the spinach in batches.

STEP 2

Return the chorizo to the skillet with the sweet potatoes and spinach. Turn the heat to medium-low and stir the contents. Add the salt and pepper and continue to stir occasionally. Cook for three to five more minutes or until all the ingredients are done to your desired tenderness.

Serve immediately with a runny egg or two if desired.

NUTRITION VALUE	817 Cal, 20g fat, 1.9g saturated fat, 13.6g fiber, 21g protein, 14g carbs.

LODGE

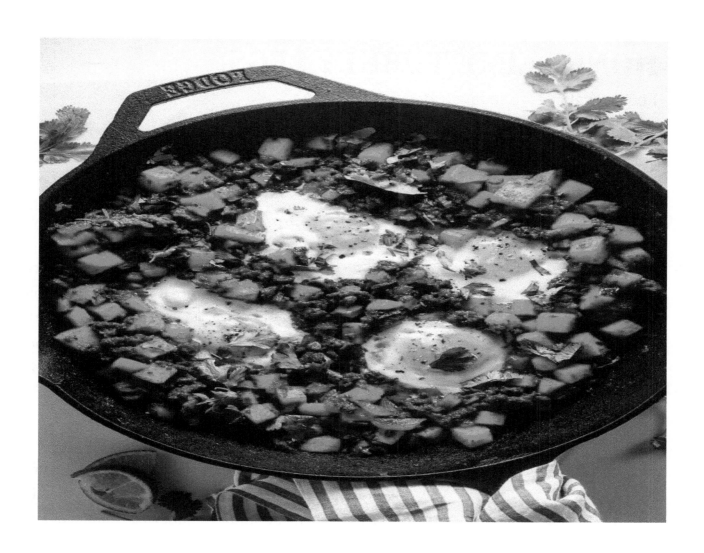

HONEY LIME TURKEY LEGS

Recipe that everyone love.

MAKES 4 SERVING/ TOTAL TIME 60 MINUTE

INGREDIENTS

Brine

4 cups Water

1/2 cup Sea salt

2 tbs Raw honey

1/2 tbs Italian seasonings

1 tsp Black pepper

Turkey legs

4 Turkey legs (large)

2 tbs olive oil

1/3 cup Lime juice (fresh squeezed)

1 tbs Raw honey

1/4 tsp Red pepper flakes

1/2 Shallot (finely minced)

2 cloves garlic (finely minced)

1/2 tsp Black pepper

Additional olive oil (for grill)

METHOD

Brine

Place all brine ingredients into a saucepan. Heat on medium-high and stir frequently until all ingredients are well-combined and mixture is reaching a low boil. Place turkey legs in a large re-sealable freezer bag. Use more than one bag if needed. Pour the brine over the turkey legs, seal the bag, and refrigerate for up to 24 hours

Turkey legs

Heat the olive oil over medium heat in a saucepan. Add the pepper flakes, garlic, and shallots, and sauté until shallots are soft. Add the lime juice, honey, and black pepper, and stir often until well-combined. Set mixture aside. Place brine-soaked turkey legs on grill. Brush with the lime honey mixture and cook for ten to twelve minutes with lid closed before turning. Turn the turkey legs and brush with lime honey mixture again. Continue to cook and brush with the lime honey mixture about every ten minutes until the legs are done Get ready to get your hands dirty and enjoy!

NUTRITION VALUE	145 Cal, 15g fat, 2g saturated fat, 1g fiber, 21g protein, 3g carbs.

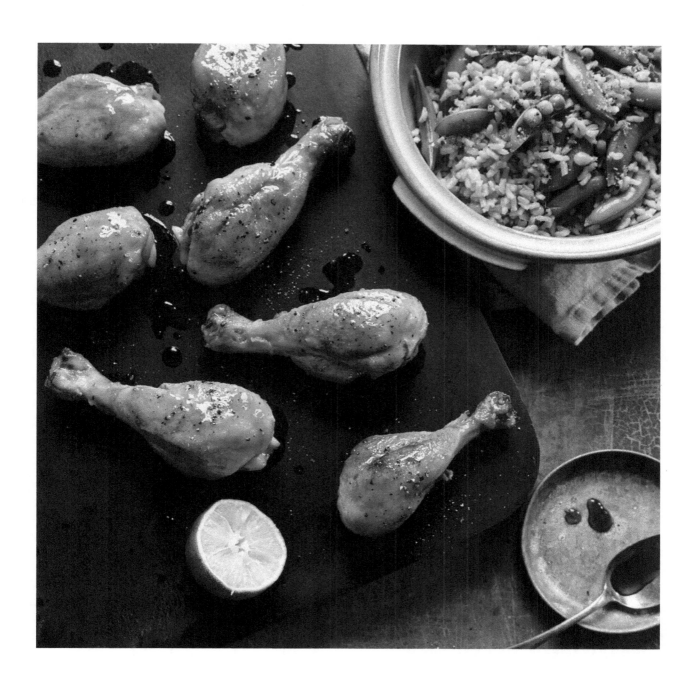

SWEET CABBAGE SALAD

Salads are a great way to pack in a load of veggies but they can get a bit same if you don't mix up the ingredients you use.

MAKES 4 SERVING/ TOTAL TIME 10 MINUTE

INGREDIENTS

Salad

1/2 Red cabbage (Head shredded)

16 oz Pineapple chunks (in 100% juice)

1/2 c Sunflower seeds

Dressing

1/2 tsp Salt

1 tsp Onion powder

1 tsp Apple cider vinegar

3 tsp EVOO

Leftover juice (from strained pineapple)

METHOD

STEP 1

Open pineapple, and strain liquid into a medium-sized Mason jar.

In a large bowl, mix the cabbage, pineapple chunks, and sunflower seeds. Blend well.

STEP 2

Add salt, onion powder, vinegar, and EVOO to the Mason jar with reserved pineapple juice. Shake well.

Drizzle cabbage salad with dressing, and store extra separately so that it doesn't make the salad soggy.

NUTRITION VALUE	273 Cal, 18g fat, 2g saturated fat, 4g fiber, 21g protein, 14g carbs.

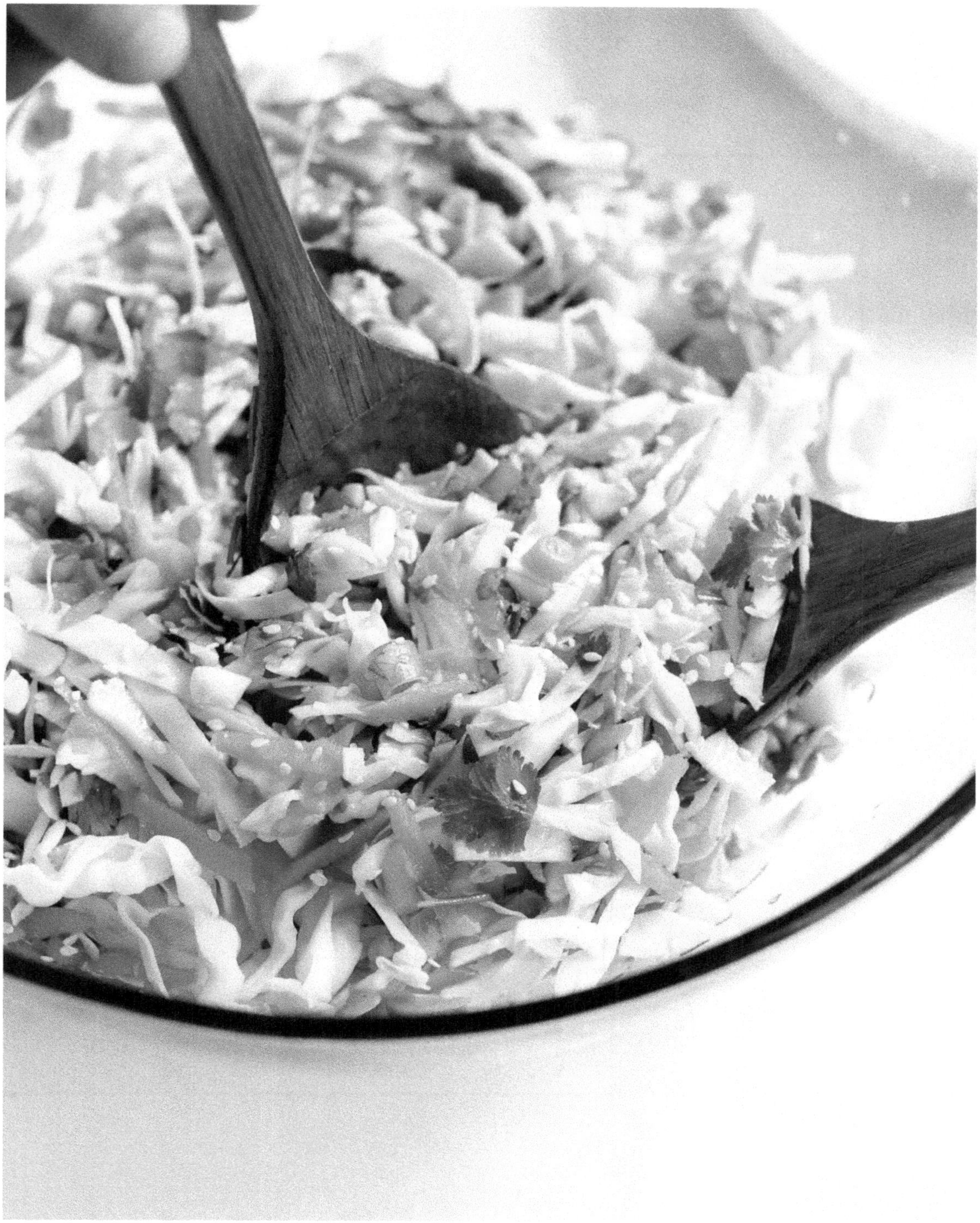

PASTRAMI WRAPS

This is a simple meal which can be used as a snack or a starter.

MAKES 2 SERVING/ TOTAL TIME 20 MINUTE

INGREDIENTS

4 oz Pastrami

1 Head green leafy lettuce (or radicchio)

8 tsp Brown mustard

30 Dill pickle chips

1/4 Purple onion (thinly sliced)

METHOD

STEP 1

Rinse and trim lettuce, and lay out flat in sheets.

Place two pieces of pastrami on each sheet of lettuce.

Top with thinly sliced onion, pickles, and half a tsp of brown mustard.

Roll, secure with toothpicks if desired, and enjoy!

NUTRITION VALUE

127 Cal, 11g fat, 2g saturated fat, 2g fiber, 23g protein, 6g carbs.

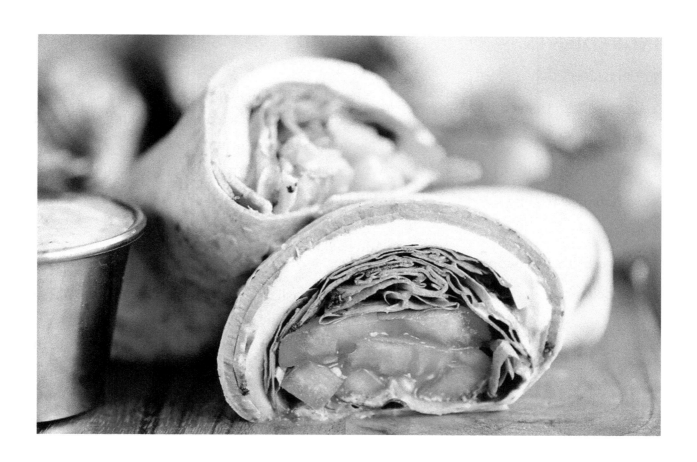

STUFFED ACORN SQUASH

Yet another delicious and filling meal that's perfect for colder weather. This is a meal that almost everyone will love. Seconds all round!

MAKES 2 SERVING/ TOTAL TIME 20 MINUTE

INGREDIENTS

1/2 lb Beef

1 Acorn squash (halved

1 tbsp garlic (minced)

1/2 Onion (small, diced)

1 tsp Italian seasoning

1 tsp Salt

1 tsp Fresh cracked pepper

1 tsp Coconut oil

METHOD

STEP 1

Preheat oven to 350 degrees.

Place squash halves face down on baking sheet, and bake for 60 minutes or until tender.

While squash is baking, warm coconut oil (or other cooking fat) in skillet. Add garlic and onion, and heat until fragrant.

Add beef to skillet, and brown.

STEP 2

Remove squash from oven, and allow to cool. Once cool, remove seeds, and discard.

Using a spoon, remove squash flesh, and add it to the skillet with the beef. Combine well.

Once the squash and beef mixture are fully combined and warmed through, use spoon to add mixture back into the squash shells.

Garnish with fresh chopped parsley.

NUTRITION VALUE	356 Cal, 20g fat, 11g saturated fat, 0.2g fiber, 31g protein, 4g carbs.

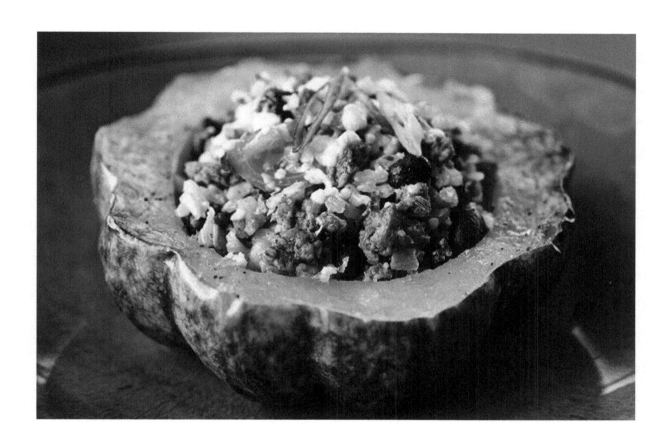

SWEET POTATO BACON EGG SALAD

This salad contains all of our favorites, and is interesting enough to tempt even the most salad-averse among us!

MAKES 2 SERVING/ TOTAL TIME 20 MINUTE

INGREDIENTS

Salad

1 Sweet potato (diced)

6 pieces bacon (chopped)

2 Eggs (hard boiled and cubed)

Dressing

1/2 c Coconut milk

1 tbsp Dill (dried)

2 tbsp Juice from 1/2 lemon

1 tbsp Yellow mustard

1/2 tsp Salt

1 tsp Onion powder

METHOD

STEP 1

Boil eggs, remove shells, and cube.

Brown bacon until crisp, and chop roughly.

Using leftover bacon fat in the pan, fry diced sweet potato until tender (about 8-10 minutes).

STEP 2

While those items are cooking, add ingredients for the dressing to a medium-sized mixing bowl, and whisk. Once everything is complete, add bacon, eggs, and potatoes to a large bowl, and combine well.

Once combined, spoon into bowls, and top with dressing mixture.

NUTRITION VALUE

142 Cal, 11g fat, 9g saturated fat, 1g fiber, 21g protein, 10 carbs.

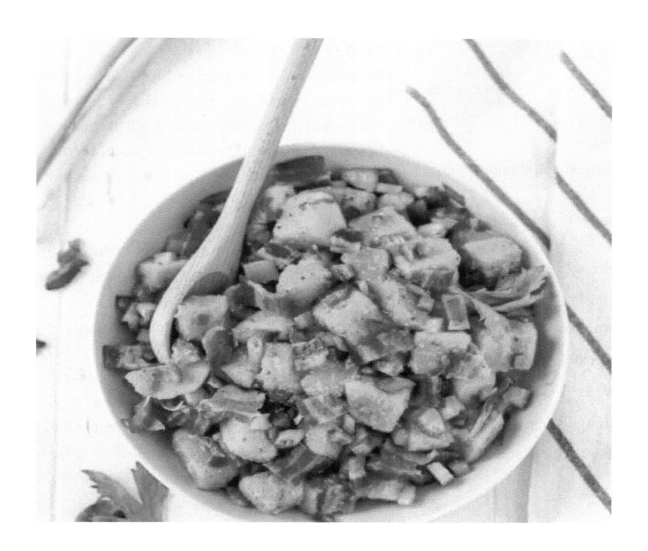

EGGS IN SPICY PALEO TOMATO SAUCE

Paleo tomato sauce is a one thing that could be undeniably a gift from heaven.

MAKES 4 SERVING/ TOTAL TIME 20 MINUTE

INGREDIENTS

2 tbsp olive oil

2 Red bell peppers (seeded and diced)

2 Jalapeño peppers (large, seeded and chopped)

1 Onion (medium, chopped (about 1 c)

5 cloves garlic (chopped (about 1.5 tbsp))

2 tsp Cumin

1/2 tbsp Salt

3 tbsp Tomato paste

1 can Tomatoes (28 oz, diced)

1/2 c Water

8 Eggs (large)

2 tbsp Parsley or cilantro (chopped)

METHOD

STEP 1

Heat oil in skillet over medium heat. Add bell peppers, jalapeños, onion, garlic, cumin, and 3/4 tsp of the salt. Cook while stirring occasionally, until the onion becomes translucent. This will take about seven minutes. Add the tomato paste to the veggies, and mix well.

STEP 2

Add tomatoes and their liquid plus 1/2 c water. Bring the mixture to a low boil. Simmer for about 7 minutes, stirring occasional, until sauce has thickened.

Using the back of a large spoon, make "pockets" in the tomato sauce for the eggs.

Carefully crack each egg into a "pocket" or crack each egg into a small cup and pour into pockets.

Cover the skillet (DO NOT STIR!) and simmer for about 8 minutes or until eggs reach your desired "done-ness".

Sprinkle eggs with remaining salt, freshly ground pepper, and chopped fresh cilantro.

NUTRITION VALUE	663 Cal, 20g fat, 12g saturated fat, 1g fiber, 61g protein, 1g carbs.

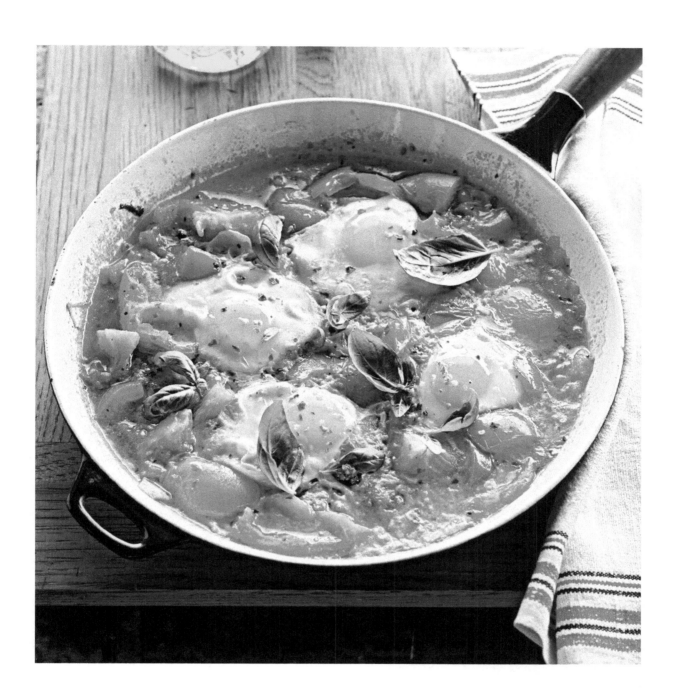

VAMPIRE CHICKEN BAKE

This is a delicious and healthy meal for all the family. Feel free to switch up the vegetables according to your own tastes.

MAKES 2 SERVING/ TOTAL TIME 60 MINUTE

INGREDIENTS

4 Boneless skinless chicken thighs

1 c Peas

1 c Cauliflower

1 1/2 tbsp garlic (minced)

1 Chopped onion (small, about 3/4 c)

2 Beets (small, cubed (about 1 c)

1 tbsp Butter

Sea salt and fresh cracked pepper (to taste)

Drizzle of EVOO

METHOD

STEP 1

Preheat oven to 350.

Drizzle olive oil in a Pyrex casserole dish. Add beets, peas, cauliflower, garlic, and onion, and mix well.

Place the tbsp of butter on top, and then add chicken thighs.

STEP 2

Add salt and cracked pepper to taste.

Cover, and bake for 45 minutes.

Remove lid, and bake for an additional 15-20 minutes, or until chicken is browned.

NUTRITION VALUE	193 Cal, 7g fat, 4g saturated fat, 9g fiber, 21g protein, 14g carbs.

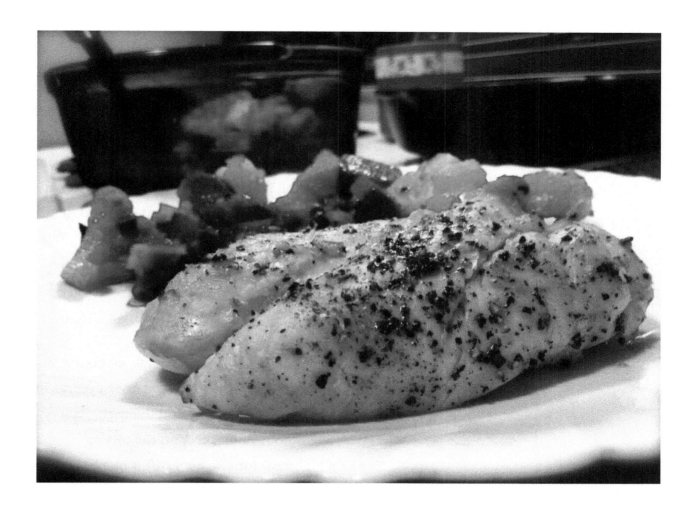

THANKSGIVING CROCK-POT TURKEY

This is our thanksgiving crockpot recipe that we would love for you to try.

MAKES 5 SERVING/ TOTAL TIME 45 MINUTE

INGREDIENTS

1 Bone-in turkey breast (get a smaller size if possible)

1 yellow onion (chopped)

1 Stalk of celery (chopped)

2 Carrots (large , peeled and chopped)

3 cloves garlic (whole)

3 tbs Onion flakes (dried)

1/2 tbs Onion powder

1/2 tbs Italian seasoning

1/2 tbs Black pepper

METHOD

STEP 1

Rinse the turkey breast off in cold water. If the breast is too large to fit in your crock pot, cut the meat from the bone into large pieces, leaving as much skin intact as possible. Mix the onion flakes, onion powder, Italian seasoning, and black pepper together. You can just put all of these ingredients into a small zip lock bag, and shake, or get all fancy with a mortar and pestle. Another (lazy) option is to use one packet of onion soup mix, but be sure to read the label, and be on the lookout for MSG, sugar, and other additives you'd prefer to avoid.
Rub the onion flake mixture into the turkey, placing as much under the skin as possible.

STEP 2

Add enough water to the crock pot to just cover the bottom. Place the turkey breast (or breast pieces if you had to cut) in the center, and add the garlic, celery, carrot, and onion chunks around the turkey.
Cook on high heat for one hour. After one hour, turn the heat down to low, and cook for an additional 7 – 8 hours or until done. Serve immediately, and save any leftovers.

NUTRITION VALUE

238 Cal, 20g fat, 15g saturated fat, 2g fiber, 21g protein, 15g carbs.

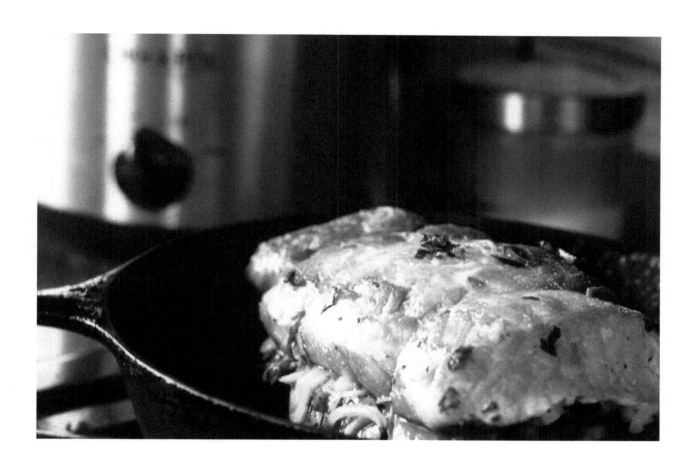

SALSA VERDE CHICKEN

Chicken is a staple in any paleo's diet, but let's not be boring here. Let's spice our meals up, and put a twist on our usual meals. This recipe will allow you to do just that. Enjoy!

MAKES 4 SERVING/ TOTAL TIME 40 MINUTE

INGREDIENTS

2 lbs Boneless skinless chicken parts (about 4 pieces)

1 can Coconut milk

2 c Green "verde" salsa

1 tsp Salt

1 tsp Onion powder

1 tsp Garlic powder

1 tsp Cumin

2 tbsp Arrowroot powder (+ 4 water)

METHOD

STEP 1

Preheat oven to 400 degrees.

Add all of the ingredients except for arrowroot and water to a large casserole baking dish.

Cover with tin foil, and bake for thirty minutes.

While baking, add arrowroot and water to a small jar with a lid. Shake well to combine. You'll probably have to do this again right before adding it to the chicken because will probably separate.

STEP 2

At the thirty minute mark, remove chicken from the oven, add the arrowroot and water mixture, and whisk into sauce, so that it is combined well.

Bake for an additional fifteen minutes.

Serve over "riced" cauliflower or lightly sautéed spinach.

NUTRITION VALUE

289 Cal, 8.7g fat, 1.9g saturated fat, 1g fiber, 59g protein, 9g carbs.

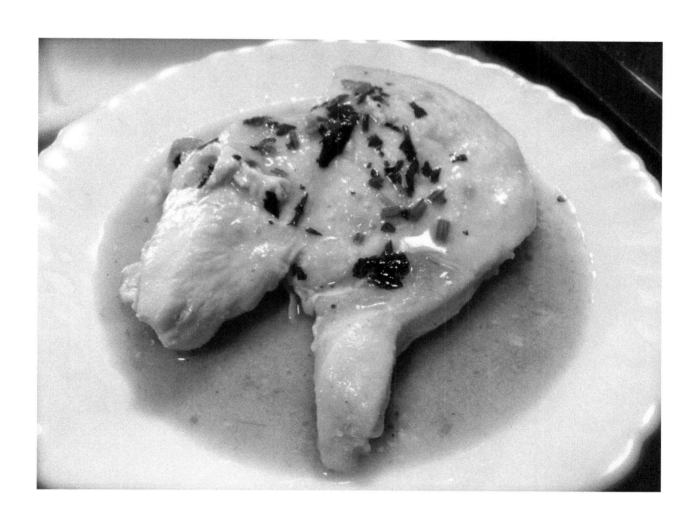

Dinner

BRILLIANT BROCCOLI SALAD

This easy raw broccoli salad is the perfect side dish for summer picnics and barbecues.

MAKES 5 SERVING/ TOTAL TIME 30 MINUTE

INGREDIENTS

2 Heads of broccoli (cut into florets)

1 Red apple (large, diced)

3/4 cup Slivered almonds

1/2 cup Raisins

3 slices bacon

For the dressing

1/4 cup Extra virgin olive oil

2 tbsp Honey

1 tbsp Dijon mustard

1 tbsp White wine vinegar

2 cloves garlic (peeled)

Juice of 1 lemon

Salt and freshly ground pepper (to taste)

METHOD

STEP 1

Cook the bacon in a skillet until crisp.

Remove from the pan to a paper towel-lined plate. Crumble and set aside.

Lightly toast the almonds in a separate skillet over medium heat until golden. Set aside to cool.

STEP 2

Place all the ingredients for the dressing into a blender or food processor and purée until smooth. Adjust salt and pepper to taste.

Add the broccoli, apple, and raisins into a large bowl and stir to combine.

Add the bacon and almonds.

Drizzle in the dressing and stir well to coat.

Refrigerate for one hour before serving.

NUTRITION VALUE

398 Cal, 20g fat, 3g saturated fat, 5g fiber, 22g protein, 14g carbs.

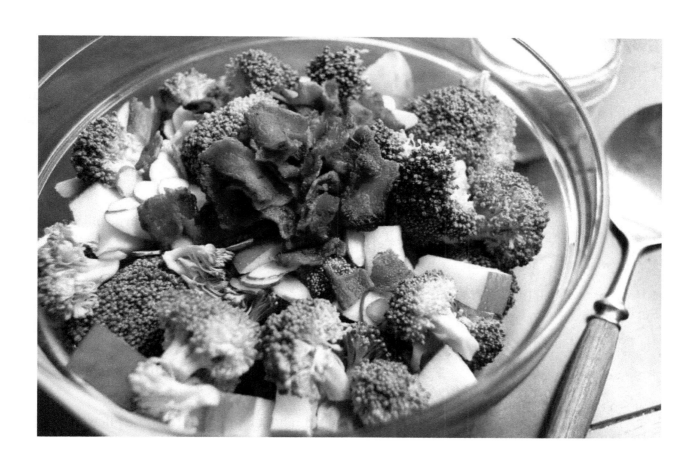

PALEO VEGETABLE CURRY

The paleo diet has plenty of vegetarian-friendly options, including this delicious, spicy curry.

MAKES 4 SERVING/ TOTAL TIME 30 MINUTE

INGREDIENTS

1 tbsp Coconut oil

2 tbsp Panaeng curry paste

1 yellow onion (medium, diced)

4 cloves garlic (minced)

1/2 Red bell pepper (thinly sliced)

1/2 yellow bell pepper (thinly sliced)

1 Yellow squash (small, chopped)

1 Head of broccoli (small, cut into florets)

1 14 oz can Coconut milk

1 tsp Coconut aminos

Salt (to taste)

2 tsp Lime juice

1/4 cup Cilantro (chopped)

METHOD

STEP 1

Melt the coconut oil in a large pan over medium heat.

Add the curry paste and cook for 2-3 minutes, stirring frequently.

Add the onion and garlic to the pan, along with a dash of salt, and sauté for 4-5 minutes.

Stir in the bell peppers, squash, and broccoli.

Sauté for 2-3 minutes more.

STEP 2

Add the coconut milk and coconut aminos to the pan and bring to a simmer.

Cook for 10-15 minutes until the coconut milk has thickened slightly and the vegetables are tender.

Adjust salt to taste.

Remove from heat and stir in the lime juice.

Top with cilantro to serve.

NUTRITION VALUE	331 Kcal, 20g fat, 5g fiber, 22g protein, 13g carbs.

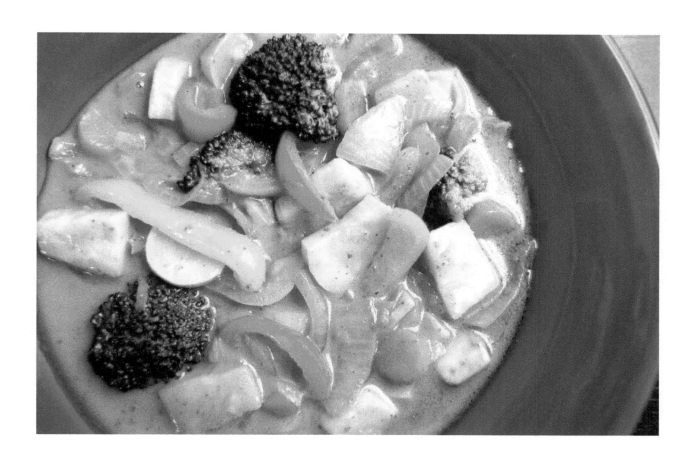

VEGETABLE SOUP WITH CABBAGE AND ONION "NOODLES"

That's a healthy bunch of ingredients. In this cuisine, you will learn how to prepare it for yourself.

MAKES 6 SERVING/ TOTAL TIME 30 MINUTE

INGREDIENTS

4 c Bone broth*

1 c White onion (very thinly sliced, use a mandolin slicer)

1 c Cabbage (very thinly sliced)

1/2 c Carrots (chopped)

1/2 c Spinach (chopped)

1 tbsp garlic (minced)

1/2 tbsp Coconut oil

Salt and pepper (to taste)

1 Bay leaf

METHOD

STEP 1

Add coconut oil and minced garlic to soup pot. Warm until fragrant.

Add bone broth to soup pot and turn up heat to bring soup to a slight simmer.

Add cabbage, onions, carrots, and bay leaf. Simmer for 20 minutes.

STEP 2

Once onions, cabbage, and carrots are fully cooked but not mushy, add in spinach. Simmer 5 minutes longer.

Taste test the soup and add salt and pepper. Remember, the bone broth has not been salted, so you might have to be generous with the salt.

Garnish with paleo-approved hot sauce.

NUTRITION VALUE	471 Cal, 20g fat, 11g saturated fat, 2g fiber, 32g protein, 14.9g carbs.

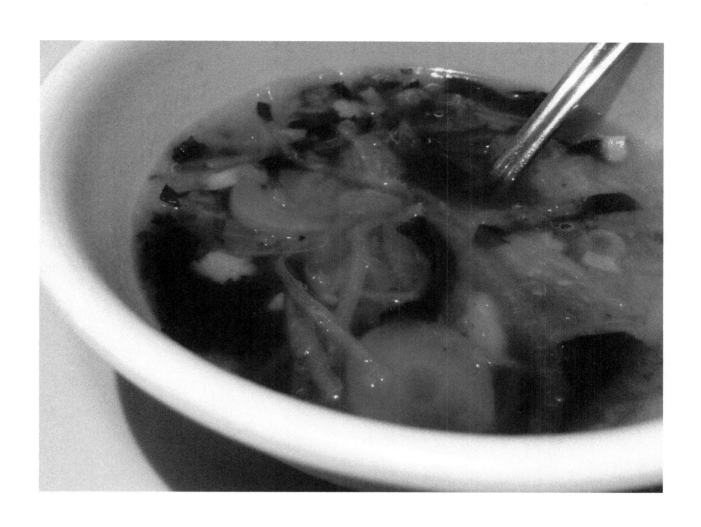

PALEO PULLED PORK & BROCCOLI

This slow cooker dish takes boring pork and turns it into an exciting dinner in just a few steps.

MAKES 4 SERVING/ TOTAL TIME 30 MINUTE

INGREDIENTS

1 lb Pork (feel free to use a cut that would be too tough to cook any other way)

1/2 c Onions (shredded)

1/2 c Cabbage (shredded)

1 tsp Garlic powder

1 tsp Onion powder

Sea salt and fresh ground pepper (to taste)

1/2 c Water

1 c Broccoli florets

Cayenne pepper (optional)

Coconut aminos (optional)

Ginger (Fresh grated - optional)

METHOD

STEP 1

Add everything but broccoli to Crock-Pot and cook on low for 8 hours or until pork falls off easily.
Once the pork is done, use 2 forks to shred the meat and mix everything together.

STEP 2

Add broccoli florets into the Crock-Pot for about 15 minutes or until they are steamed and warmed through. Garnish with cayenne pepper, coconut aminos, and fresh grated ginger.

NUTRITION VALUE

355 Cal, 19g fat, 7g saturated fat, 3g fiber, 34g protein, 10g carbs.

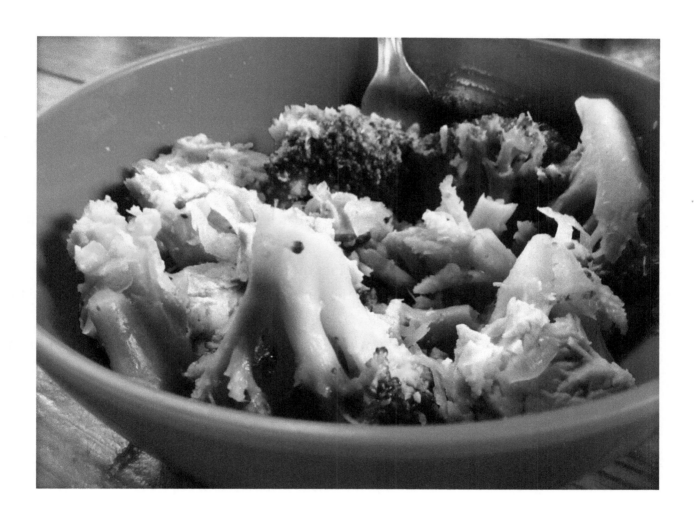

SLOW COOKER BALSAMIC SHORT RIBS

This Is The Short Ribs Slow Cooker With Balsamic Vinegar Recipe.

MAKES 4 SERVING/ TOTAL TIME 35 MINUTE

INGREDIENTS

2.5 lbs Bone-in beef short ribs

1-2 tbsp Coconut oil

1 15- oz can Tomato sauce

1/2 cup Balsamic vinegar

1 tbsp Honey

6 cloves garlic (smashed)

For the dry rub

2 tbsp Salt

1 tbsp Rosemary (dried)

1 tbsp Thyme (dried)

2 tsp Garlic powder

1 tsp Onion powder

1 tsp Smoked paprika

1 tsp Freshly ground pepper

METHOD

STEP 1

In a small bowl, stir together all of the ingredients for the spice rub.

Pat the short ribs dry with a paper towel and rub generously with the spice mixture.

Melt the coconut oil in a large skillet over medium-high heat.

STEP 2

Working in batches, sear the short ribs for 2-3 minutes per side.

Place into the slow cooker.

Add the tomato sauce, balsamic, honey, and garlic to the slow cooker with the short ribs.

Cover and cook on low heat for 5-6 hours until the beef is tender.

Serve warm.

NUTRITION VALUE	646 Cal, 20g fat, 14g saturated fat, 4g fiber, 46g protein, 11g carbs.

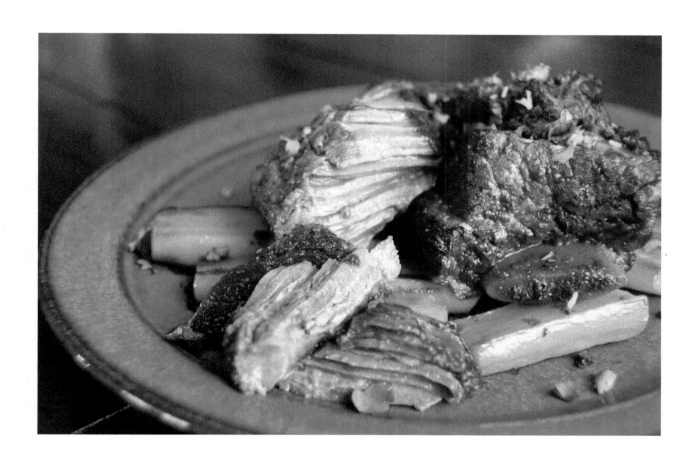

CHICKEN WITH ROSEMARY MUSHROOM SAUCE

Tender chicken is smothered with a gravy-like mushroom sauce in this meal that is ready in no time.

MAKES 2 SERVING/ TOTAL TIME 30 MINUTE

INGREDIENTS

1 lb Skinless chicken thighs and legs

Salt and pepper (to taste)

2 tbsp Extra virgin olive oil (divided)

1/2 yellow onion (sliced)

2 cloves garlic (minced)

1 tbsp Fresh rosemary (chopped)

6 oz White mushrooms (sliced)

2-3 tbsp Coconut milk

1/4 cup Chicken broth

METHOD

STEP 1

Generously season the chicken with salt and pepper. Heat one tablespoon of olive oil in a large skillet over medium-high heat. Add the chicken and sear on both sides until completely browned and cooked through. Remove, put on a plate, and set aside.

In the same skillet, heat the remaining tablespoon of olive oil. Add the onion, garlic, and rosemary to the pan and sauté for 4-5 minutes.

Add the mushrooms and cook for another 5 minutes until browned.

STEP 2

Pour in the chicken broth and coconut milk and stir to combine, scraping any browned pieces off the bottom of the pan.

Bring to a boil, then reduce the heat and simmer for 4-5 minutes until the sauce thickens.

Add salt and pepper to taste.

If desired, purée the sauce in a blender until smooth.

Serve warm sauce drizzled over the seared chicken.

NUTRITION VALUE	205 Cal, 19g fat, 5g saturated fat, 4g fiber, 22g protein, 8g carbs.

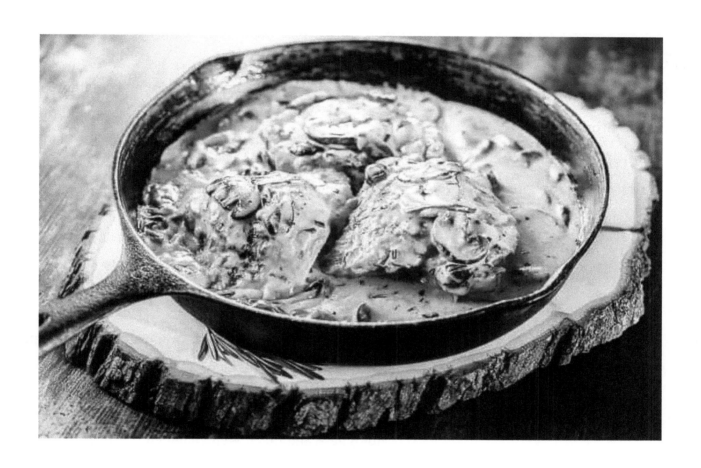

GRILLED EGGPLANT WITH PORK & MINT BOLOGNESE

This Dish Is Super Easy To Prepare, Yet It Has A Unique Combo Of Flavors, So It'll Feel Like A Fun New Treat! This Is Going On My Short List Of Standby Dinners For Sure!

MAKES 4 SERVING/ TOTAL TIME 40 MINUTE

INGREDIENTS

1 Eggplant (large)

1/2 lb Ground pork

1 cn Tomatoes (diced, about 2 c)

1 c Mint (freshly chopped)

1/2 c Onions (diced)

3 tbsp garlic (minced)

2 c Mushroom (canned)

3 tbsp Sea salt

1 tbsp Coconut oil

METHOD

Peel the skin off the entire eggplant and cut it into discs that are about 1/4 inch thick. Place the eggplant discs into large serving bowl and cover them evenly and liberally with 3 tbsp sea salt. This will remove the bitter flavor that is normally associated with eggplant.

Set the eggplant aside for 30 minutes to an hour, so that the sea salt can "pull" the bitterness out. While the eggplant is in the brine, add coconut oil to a large saucepan and sauté the onions and garlic until they are translucent and fragrant.

Add the ground pork into the onion and garlic mix and brown it. Once the meat is brown, add in the diced onions and mushrooms. Warm them through and turn down the heat to low. Add fresh chopped mint to the Bolognese and mix it well. Using your grill, grill each slice of eggplant for about 5-7 minutes or until it is soft yet firm . Once you've grilled the eggplant, lay 2-3 discs on each plate and top with pork and mint Bolognese. Then garnish the dish with fresh chopped mint.

NUTRITION VALUE

233 Cal, 16g fat, 8g saturated fat, 2g fiber, 21g protein, 14g carbs.

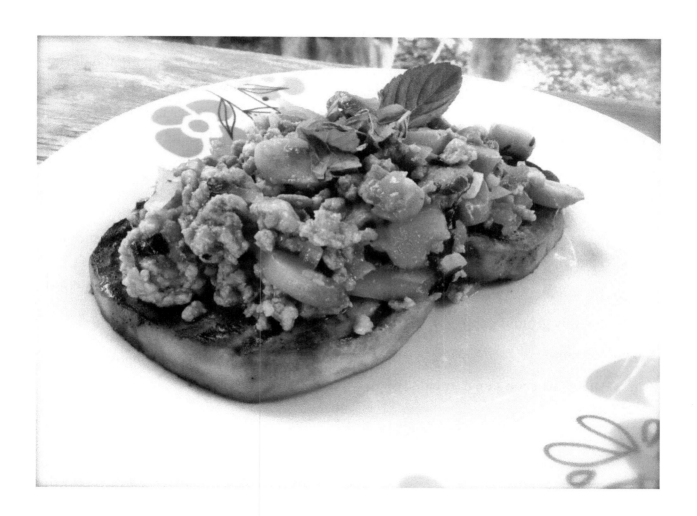

SCRUMMY BARBECUE PORK

Sweet, tangy barbecue pork is easy to make in the slow cooker. You simply place the pork into the pot and leave it to cook for most of the day.

MAKES 6 SERVING/ TOTAL TIME 40 MINUTE

INGREDIENTS

3 lbs Pork shoulder

1 White onion (medium, diced)

For the spice rub

2 tbsp Chili powder

1 1/2 tsp Salt

1 tsp Onion powder

1 tsp Cumin

1 tsp Oregano (dried)

1/2 tsp Coriander

1/2 tsp Freshly ground pepper

1/4 tsp Cayenne

2 cups Paleo barbecue sauce (divided)

METHOD

STEP 1

Add the onion into the Crock-Pot. Combine the ingredients for the spice rub in a small bowl. Pat the pork shoulder dry with a paper towel. Rub the spice mixture into the pork and set into the Crock-Pot. Drizzle with 1 cup of the barbecue sauce. Cover and cook on low heat for 7-8 hours.

STEP 2

Remove the pork from the Crock-Pot and shred. Strain any of the liquid remaining in the slow cooker through a fine mesh strainer or cheesecloth. Place the pork back into the empty Crock-Pot, along with the remaining cup of barbecue sauce. Pour in 1/4-1/2 cup of the strained liquid and stir. Cook on low for an additional 30 minutes. Serve warm.

NUTRITION VALUE

80 Cal, 3g fat, 0.4g saturated fat, 3g fiber, 24g protein, 14g carbs.

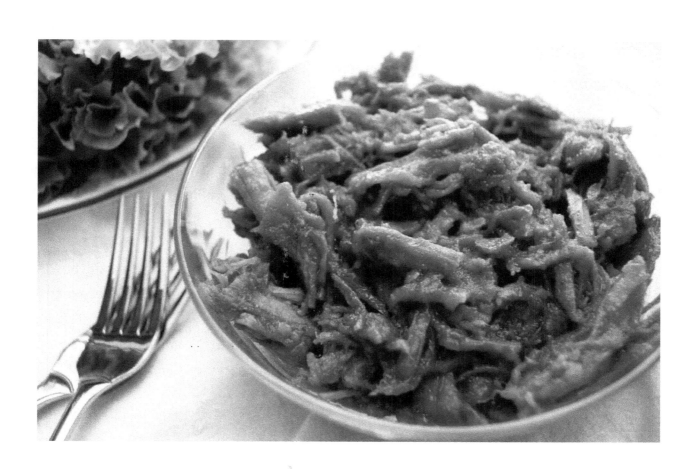

JALAPEÑO AND APPLE COLESLAW

Jalapeno coleslaw is a salad of different vegetables and fruit like carrots, cabbage, and green apples that makes it very healthy.

MAKES 6 SERVING/ TOTAL TIME 20 MINUTE

INGREDIENTS

4 c Cabbage (shredded)

1 Green apple (thinly sliced)

1 Carrot (thinly sliced)

1/2 in Red onion (thinly sliced rings)

1 Fresh jalapeño (diced, with seeds and ribs removed)

2 tbsp Apple cider vinegar

1 tbsp EVOO

1/2 tsp Salt

1/2 tsp Freshly ground pepper

METHOD

STEP 1

Shred cabbage and add to large mixing bowl.

Add shredded apple, carrot, and onion to the cabbage. Toss.

Remove ribs and seeds from jalapeño and dice. I diced mine into large chunks because I wanted people who didn't like jalapeño to be able to pick it out. Add jalapeño to bowl.

STEP 2

Add vinegar, olive oil, salt, and pepper to the bowl. Combine well so that all the ingredients get a nice coating of the dressing.

Allow flavors to soak into the mix in the fridge for a couple hours before serving.

NUTRITION VALUE

822 Cal, 19g fat, 1.9g saturated fat, 10g fiber, 20g protein, 13g carbs.

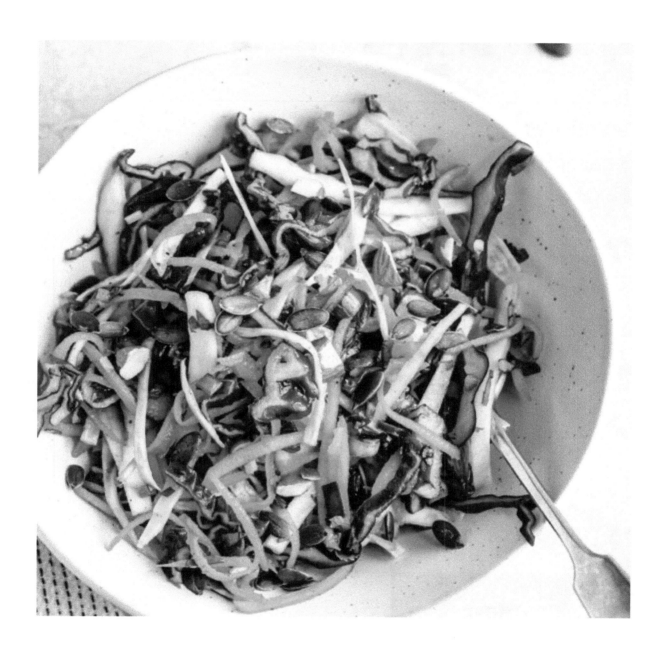

BONFIRE-ROASTED VEGGIES

These bonfire veggie packets are so easy and delicious that you'll want to eat them every night of the week!

MAKES 2 SERVING/ TOTAL TIME 10 MINUTE

INGREDIENTS

2 c Zucchini (thickly chopped)

1 c Onion (diced)

1/2 c Fresh mushrooms (sliced)

1/2 c Red pepper (diced)

2 tbsp Butter

Dash of garlic powder

Dash of onion powder

Sea salt and freshly ground pepper (to taste)

Tin foil

METHOD

STEP 1

Lay out 2 sheets of tin foil (about 12 inches by 12 inches).

Divide the veggies into groups, and portion them out on each sheet of tin foil.

Sprinkle each veggie packet with seasonings and add 1 tbsp butter to each packet.

STEP 2

Carefully fold and roll up the veggies in the tin foil. I recommend wrapping the packets with a second sheet of tin foil before roasting; this will help keep everything together and keep the butter from leaking out.

Roast on a grill or bonfire for about 5 minutes on each side.

Cut open the packets

NUTRITION VALUE	207 Cal, 13g fat, 8g saturated fat, 6g fiber, 21g protein, 14g carbs.

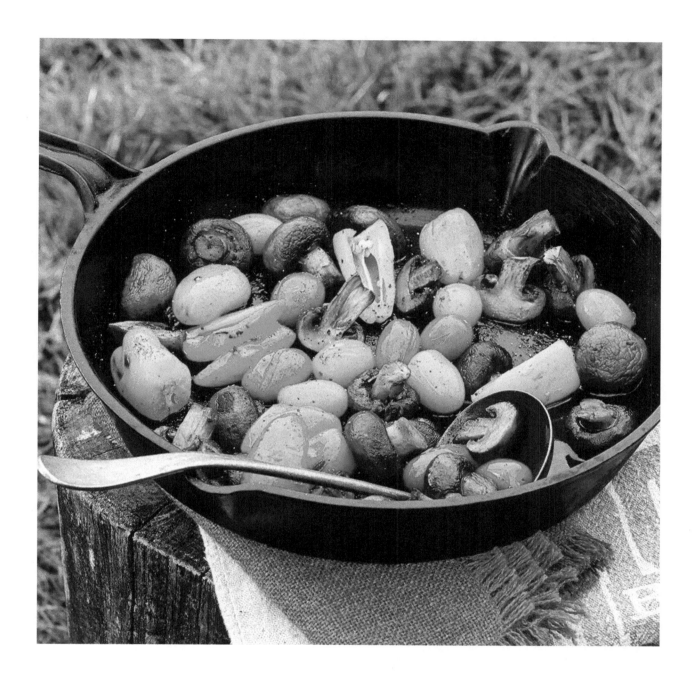

GRILLED SKIN ON FISH

There are many health benefits of eating fish. Its Omega-3 fatty acids in particular are good for your heart.

MAKES 4 SERVING/ TOTAL TIME 20 MINUTE

INGREDIENTS

8 White fish fillets (small-medium- I used yellow fin tuna and red snappert hey should be de-scaled and de-headed)

1/4 c Softened butter

1/4 c garlic (minced)

Salt and pepper (to taste)

2 Lemons

METHOD

STEP 1

Take de-scaled and de-headed fish fillets and cut flesh to the spine at a 45-degree angle from tip to tail and vice versa, creating Xs on both sides (see photo).

Mix together softened butter and minced garlic.

Using a spatula, evenly spread garlic butter on all sides of the fish, making sure to fill each of the crevices with as much tasty garlic butter as possible.

STEP 2

Heat grill to medium heat.

Place fish on grill and grill for about 3-5 minutes on each side, until flesh is flaky and white to the bone.

Serve with lemon wedges, and garnish with a sprinkle of dried dill if desired.

NUTRITION VALUE

245 Kcal, 18g fat, 3g fiber, 20g protein, 15g carbs.

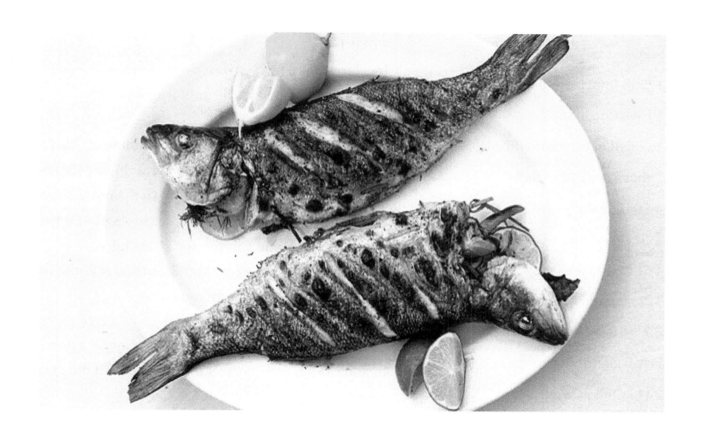

CHORIZO STEW WITH POACHED EGG

This concoction packs a punch with the many flavors it brings together.

MAKES 4 SERVING/ TOTAL TIME 30 MINUTE

INGREDIENTS

Stew

1/2 lb Chorizo sausage (clean)

1 tbsp Coconut oil

1/2 Onion (medium diced)

2 tbsp garlic (minced)

4 Stalks celery (diced)

1 can Tomato (diced)

1/2 c Cabbage (shredded)

1/2 c Spinach (chopped)

2.5 c Bone broth*

Fresh cilantro (chopped)

1 tsp Chili powder

1/2 tsp Smoked paprika

Salt and pepper (to taste)

Poached eggs

3 c Water

A dash of vinegar

4 Eggs

METHOD
STEP 1
In a large soup pot (or Dutch oven), warm coconut oil and heat onion and garlic until fragrant and transparent.

Cut chorizo into small bites or, depending on the form it comes in, remove the casing and crumble it into the pot. Chop celery and cabbage and add to the pot. Stir well.

Add one can of diced tomatoes, seasonings, and bone broth. Mix well and simmer for 20 minutes.

While stew is simmering, heat 3 c of water along with a dash of vinegar in a pot on the stove.

STEP 2
Crack eggs into individual ramekins. Now is a good time to add the spinach to the stew pot and turn down the heat.

Just as the water for the eggs is coming to a boil, gently drop one egg into the water (do this one at a time) and allow it to poach in the boiling water for approximately 2-3 minutes. Repeat for remaining eggs.

Spoon stew into bowls and top gently with poached egg. Garnish with fresh chopped cilantro.

NUTRITION VALUE	212 Cal, 18g fat, 8g saturated fat, 2g fiber, 21g protein, 7g carbs.

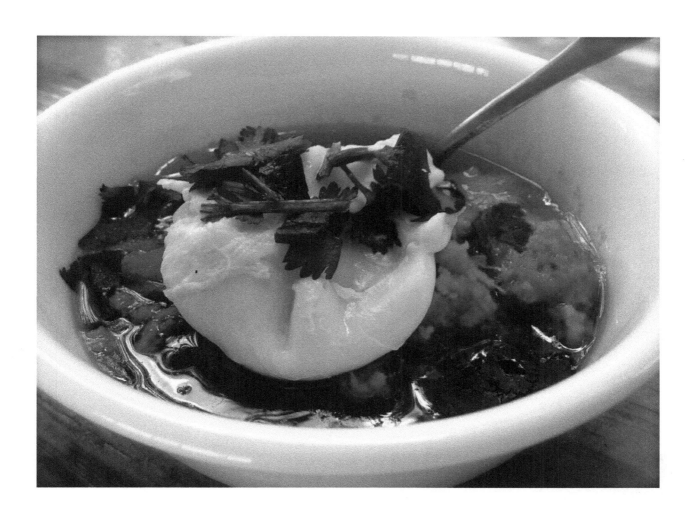

GINGER BEEF SPINACH SALAD

If you're looking for a filling but fresh and healthy meal this holiday season, this salad will sort you out.

MAKES 4 SERVING/ TOTAL TIME 10 MINUTE

INGREDIENTS

1 lb Ground beef

1 Shallot (minced)

5-6 cloves garlic (minced)

2 inches fresh ginger (minced)

1 tsp Red pepper (crushed)

1 tsp Honey

2 tbsp Coconut amino acid

Drizzle of sesame oil

4 tbsp Pineapple (crushed)

METHOD

STEP 1

Brown beef in a skillet on med-high. If desired, drain off excess fat.

Add shallot, garlic, ginger, and crushed red pepper. Cook on med high, or until the shallot becomes translucent, for about 3-4 minutes.

STEP 2

Drizzle meat with honey, sesame oil, and coconut amino acids, and mix well. Let this to cook for 2-3 more minutes to allow the flavors to combine.

Serve on top of a fresh bed of baby spinach, and garnish with 1 tbsp crushed pineapple on each salad.

NUTRITION VALUE

331 Cal, 20g fat, 8g saturated fat, 2g fiber, 29g protein, 4g carbs.

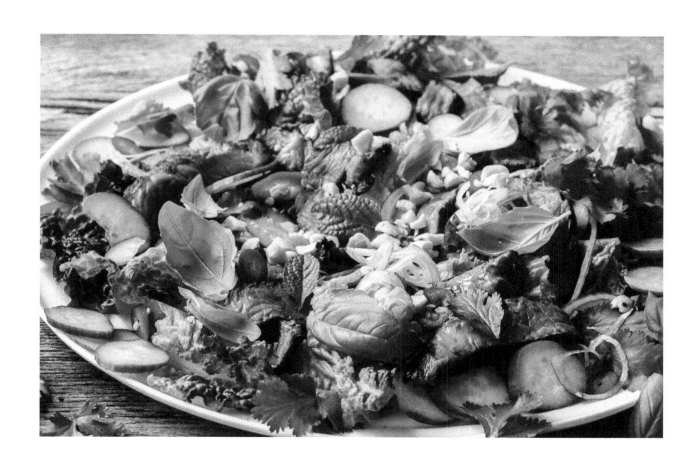

CREAMY TOMATO CHICKEN SOUP IN THE CROCK-POT

This is a really healthy meal that will fill you up and satisfy your taste buds.

MAKES 8 SERVING/ TOTAL TIME 60 MINUTE

INGREDIENTS

3 Boneless skinless chicken breasts

3 tbsp garlic (diced, adjust to taste)

1 tbsp Italian seasonings (dried, watch out for nasty additives and make sure it is "clean")

1 can Full fat coconut milk

1 can Tomatoes (diced, sugar free)

2 c Bone broth* (recipe at https://ultimatepaleoguide.com/super-easy-bone-broth-crockpot/)

1 Bay leaf

1 tbsp Butter

METHOD

STEP 1

Add everything to the Crock-Pot, and stir so that the seasonings are evenly distributed.
Cook on low for nine hours or high for six hours.

STEP 2

When it is done cooking, the chicken should fall apart easily. Use tongs to remove the chicken from the Crock-Pot, and shred it using two forks.
Add the chicken back to the soup, and mix well.

NUTRITION VALUE

175 Cal, 17g fat, 15g saturated fat, 2g fiber, 21g protein, 5g carbs.

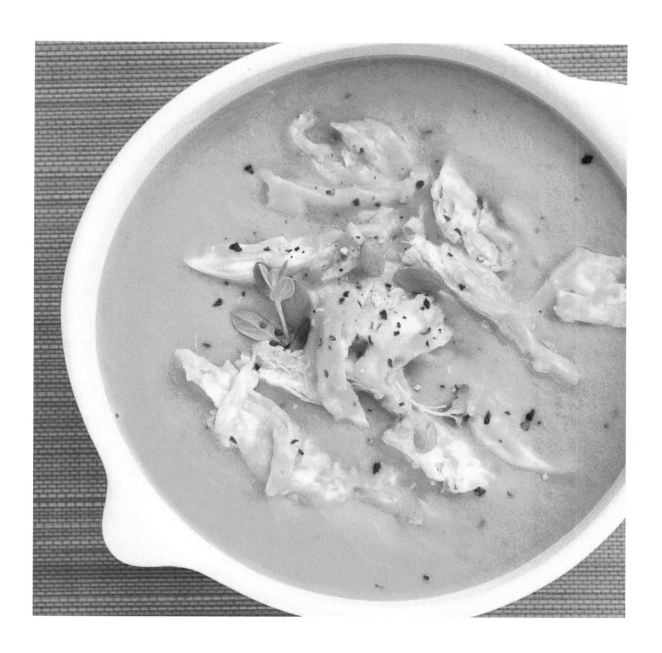

SPICY CHORIZO SOUP

Recipe that everyone love.

MAKES 4 SERVING/ TOTAL TIME 40 MINUTE

INGREDIENTS

1 Onion (medium, diced)

2 Heads of garlic (minced (about 1/2 c))

12 ounces of "clean" chorizo sausage/other spicy sausage

3 Stalks celery (diced)

1 White potato (medium, cubed)

32 oz Chicken broth

1/2 tbsp Red pepper flakes (crushed)

1/2 c Zucchini (cubed)

1/2 c Yellow squash (cubed)

Coconut oil

METHOD

STEP 1

Add a tbsp or two of coconut oil to sauté onions and garlic in a large Dutch oven or other sturdy soup pot. Sauté onions and garlic on medium-high until the onions are translucent.

Remove chorizo from its casing, and add it to the onions and garlic to brown.

Chop celery and potato while chorizo is browning.

Once diced, add celery and potato to the soup pot. Mix well.

STEP 2

Add chicken broth to the mix, along with red pepper flakes.

Allow to simmer on medium-high for about 20 minutes or until potatoes are almost done.

At the last minute, add cubed zucchini and squash, and lightly simmer for another 5-10 minutes.

Serve, and garnish with additional red pepper flakes and/or chives.

NUTRITION VALUE	269 Cal, 19g fat, 8g saturated fat, 1g fiber, 21g protein, 10g carbs.

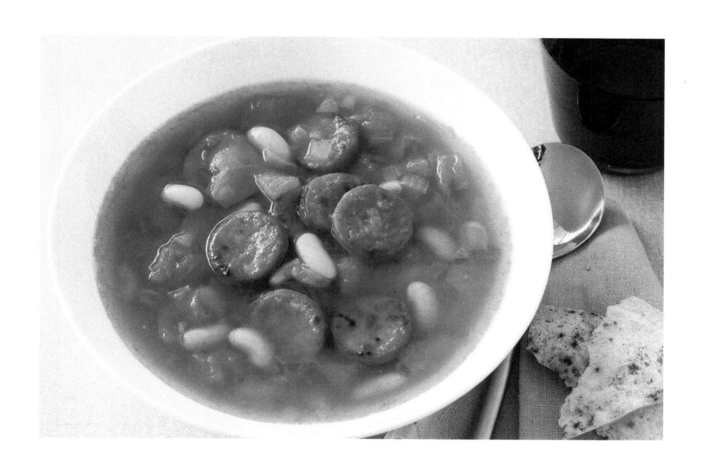

Desserts

PALEO SNICKERDOODLES

It's a to die for dessert, a chance to get the kids involved, and a way to prove to your friends that paleo tastes good!

MAKES 2 SERVING/ TOTAL TIME 40 MINUTE

INGREDIENTS

1.5 c Almond flour

2 tbsp Coconut flour

1/3 c Honey

1/3 cup Coconut oil (at room temp)

1 Egg (at room temp)

1 tsp Baking soda

1/2 tsp Salt

1/8 c Coconut Palm Sugar (for coating (optional))

1/2 tbsp Cinnamon (for coating)

METHOD

STEP 1

Pre-heat oven to 350 degrees.

In a small dish, mix together coconut palm sugar and cinnamon. Combine well and set aside.

In a large bowl, mix together coconut oil and honey. Once they are well combined, add in egg.

Finally, add in the dry ingredients. Place batter in the fridge for 5 minutes to allow for easier handling of the cookie dough.

STEP 2

Line baking sheet with parchment paper. Using hands, form balls from the cookie dough and dip one side into the coconut sugar and cinnamon mixture. Place on parchment paper and flatten slightly. You may need to rinse your hands in cold water every 3 cookies or so to allow for easier handling and less stickiness. Repeat until all batter is gone. Bake for 8 minutes at 350. Remove from oven and let cookies cool for a few minutes before transferring to a cooling rack.

NUTRITION VALUE

817 Cal, 20g fat, 1.9g saturated fat, 13.6g fiber, 21g protein, 14g carbs.

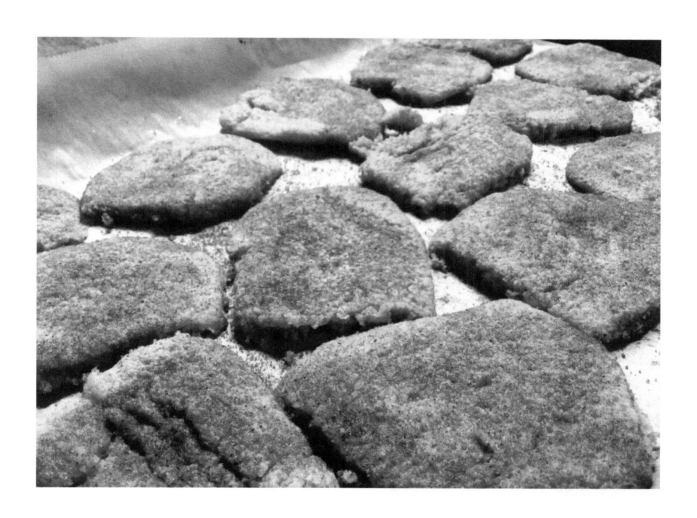

QUICK 'N' EASY FRUIT DIP

Quick 'n' Easy Fruit Dip is seriously simple to make and can be used for snacks or as part of a dessert.

MAKES 1 SERVING/ TOTAL TIME 10 MINUTE

INGREDIENTS

1 c Coconut milk

1 tsp Vanilla

2 Ripe bananas

2 tsp Coconut flour

METHOD

STEP 1

Place all ingredients in your food processor or blender. Blend until smooth.

Pour into dish and refrigerate for thirty minutes. This allows the dip to thicken.

Serve with fresh fruit.

NUTRITION VALUE	114 Cal, 11g fat, 9g saturated fat, 1g fiber, 1g protein, 4g carbs.

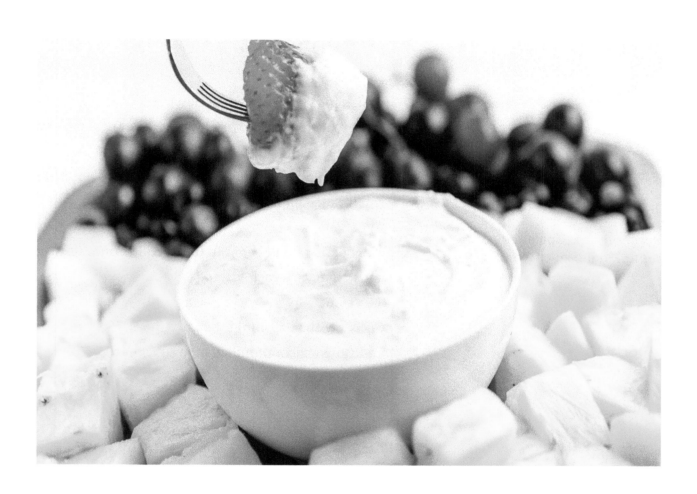

PERFECT PALEO PORRIDGE

Porridge, with its thickness and warmth, is a great way to start a cold morning.

MAKES 1 SERVING/ TOTAL TIME 10 MINUTE

INGREDIENTS

4 Eggs

2 tbsp Coconut flour

1/2 c Raisins

1/2 c Coconut milk

1 pinch Salt

Seasoning of choice (cinnamon, pumpkin pie spice, vanilla, etc.)

METHOD

STEP 1

Whisk four eggs in a small bowl.

Once whisked, add coconut flour, coconut milk, and salt. Mix well.

Once combined, bring to medium heat (do not boil) in a small sauce pan, stirring constantly.

STEP 2

The porridge will begin to thicken. Stir until desired consistency is reached.

Serve hot.

Garish with seasonings, banana slices, fresh fruit, additional coconut milk, Paleo Granola*, or Crock-Pot Fig Apple Butter

NUTRITION VALUE

638 Cal, 20g fat, 11g saturated fat, 16g fiber, 21g protein, 14g carbs.

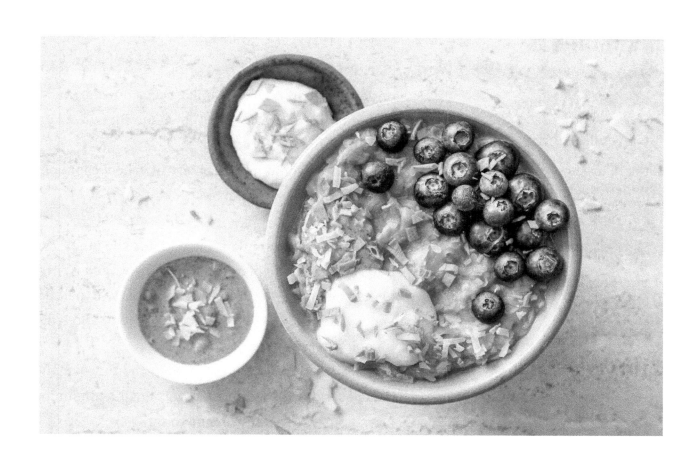

DARK CHOCOLATE MOUSSE

This chocolate mousse with a lovely texture and added fruit for extra sweetness, this treat makes for a perfect evening treat.

MAKES 4 SERVING/ TOTAL TIME 35 MINUTE

INGREDIENTS

2 Eggs

1/4 c Pure maple syrup

1 tsp Vanilla extract

2 tbsp Dark chocolate cocoa powder (unsweetened)

1/3 c Dark chocolate chips (optional)

3/4 c Coconut milk

1 pint Raspberries (or other fresh fruit)

METHOD

STEP 1

Add eggs, maple syrup, vanilla, cocoa powder, and optional chocolate chips to a blender. Blend well until combined.

Bring the coconut milk to a very high heat (not boiling) in a saucepan on the stove.

STEP 2

Once the coconut milk is hot, add it to the other ingredients in the blender in a slow and steady stream, while blending everything on low. This will melt the chocolate chips (if you opted to use them) and will "cook" the raw eggs.

Once everything is combined, pour the chocolate into small serving dishes and refrigerate for a minimum of two hours, so that it has time to set.

Serve with fresh raspberries or other fresh fruit of choice.

NUTRITION VALUE	274 Cal, 17g fat, 12g saturated fat, 12g fiber, 21g protein, 14g carbs.

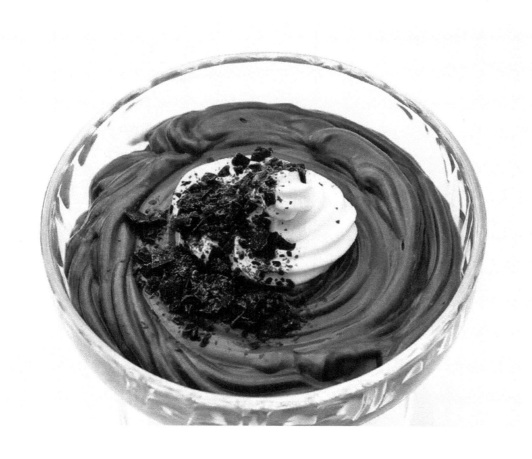

PALEO BUTTER BISCUITS

These baked treats will satisfy your sweet tooth, and may well convince all of your friends that paleo isn't so bad!

MAKES 4 SERVING/ TOTAL TIME 60 MINUTE

INGREDIENTS

2 c Almond flour

3 tbsp Coconut flour

1/4 c Butter

3 Eggs (whisked)

1/2 tsp Baking soda

1/4 tsp Salt

2 tbsp Organic coconut sugar (optional)

METHOD

STEP 1

Preheat oven to 350 degrees.

Add all the dry ingredients to a medium sized mixing bowl. Combine well with a fork.

Whisk eggs in another bowl, and add to dry ingredients.

Pour warm (not hot) melted butter into bowl. Combine well.

STEP 2

Lay out parchment paper on a large cookie sheet.

Use a large spoon or ice-cream scoop to scoop batter onto cookie sheet. Use the bottom of a glass to flatten the batter into desired shape. It helps if you rinse the bottom of the glass with cool water every time you press down on a biscuit to prevent sticking.

Bake for about fifteen minutes or until lightly golden brown.

NUTRITION VALUE

848 Cal, 20g fat, 14g saturated fat, 19g fiber, 27g protein, 14g carbs.

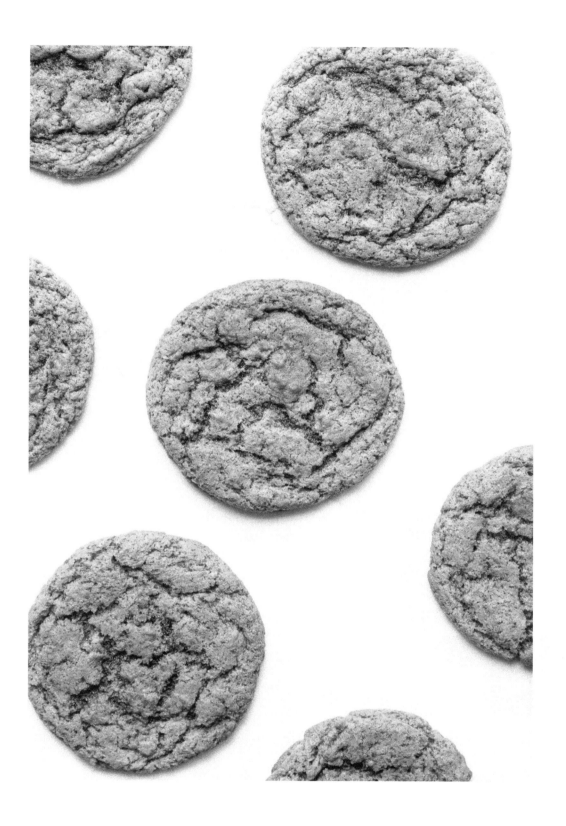

BACON CHOCOLATE CHIP COOKIES

Recipes that everyone love.

MAKES 2 SERVING/ TOTAL TIME 20 MINUTE

INGREDIENTS

2 c Almond flour

1/4 tsp Salt

1/4 tsp Baking soda

6 tbsp Coconut oil (melted)

4 tbsp Honey

2 tsp Vanilla extract

2 tbsp Coconut milk

4-6 tbsp bacon (cooked and crumbled)

1/2 c Chocolate chips

METHOD
STEP 1

Preheat oven to 350 degrees F, and line a cookie sheet with parchment paper.

In a bowl, combine all the dry ingredients, and mix well with a fork.

In another bowl, combine all the wet ingredients. Please note that the coconut oil should be melted.

Mix the wet and dry ingredients, and gently fold in the bacon crumbles. Be careful not to over-stir – stir just enough to mix well.

STEP 2

Using wet or damp hands, dig into the cookie mixture, and form small cookie balls. Gently place the cookies on the parchment-lined sheet.

These will not spread out much, so the cookies can be placed fairly close together.

Bake for 8-10 minutes, or until lightly browned on top.

NUTRITION VALUE

331 Kcal, 20g fat,
5g fiber, 22g protein, 13g carbs.

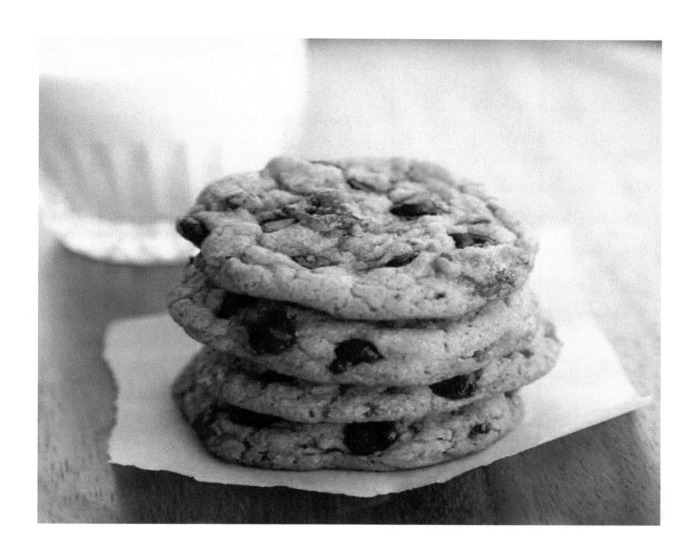

SILVER DOLLAR HOT CAKES

Recipe that everyone love.

MAKES 4 SERVING/ TOTAL TIME 70 MINUTE

INGREDIENTS

2 Eggs

3 tbsp Full fat coconut milk

1/2 tbsp Ripe banana (Mashed, or 3 unsweetened applesauce)

1/2 tsp Apple cider vinegar

1/2 tsp Vanilla extract

1.5 tbsp Coconut flour

1/4 tsp Baking soda

Pinch of salt

Powdered Stevia to taste (to taste)

Coconut oil (for frying)

METHOD

STEP 1

Put a dab of coconut oil into a pan for frying, and heat it at just under medium heat. Getting the temperature right in this recipe is the trickiest part since you want the hot cakes to cook evenly. I recommend making a few tiny hot cakes to be nibbled on during cooking at the start until you get the heat exact.

STEP 2

Mix together all other ingredients in a bowl.

Pour batter into the pan in the size of silver dollars.

Cook about 1-2 minutes on each side. You'll know it's time to flip them when little holes appear over 75% of the hot cake.

Top with butter, fresh fruit compote, whipped coconut cream, or your favorite garnish.

NUTRITION VALUE

145 Cal, 15g fat, 2g saturated fat, 1g fiber, 21g protein, 3g carbs.

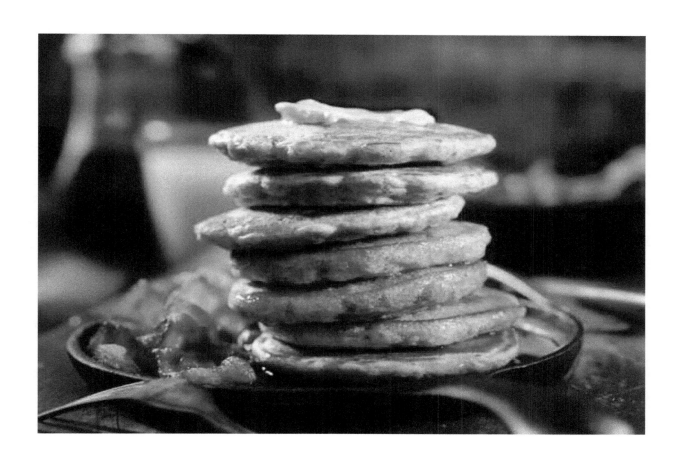

BANANA NUT BREAD

Recipe that everyone love.

MAKES 4 SERVING/ TOTAL TIME 2 HOUR

INGREDIENTS

3/4 c Coconut flour

1/4 c Arrowroot powder

1/2 c Almond flour

2 tsp Cinnamon

2 tsp Baking soda

1/4 tsp Sea salt

1/2 c Chopped pecans

1/2 c Raisins

2 Ripe bananas (medium)

3 Eggs

1/2 c Coconut milk

1 1/2 c Unsweetened apple sauce

1 tsp Vanilla

1/2 c Mixed nuts (for top)

METHOD

STEP 1

Preheat oven to 350 degrees.

Line a 9 x 5 inch bread pan with parchment paper. You'll be glad you did.

Combine all dry ingredients in a mixing bowl, and stir well with a fork.

Put all wet ingredients into a bowl, and mix well. A hand mixer works best for this with the bananas. You might also want to break the bananas into pieces instead of adding them to the bowl whole.

STEP 2

Combine both wet and dry ingredients, and mix well using a hand mixer. The batter will be dense.

Pour batter into 9 x 5 bread pan, and sprinkle the top with mixed nuts.

Bake for 60-70 minutes, or until a toothpick comes out clean.

Toast, and serve topped with almond butter.

NUTRITION VALUE

600 Cal, 20g fat, 1.9g saturated fat, 13.6g fiber, 7g protein, 14g carbs.

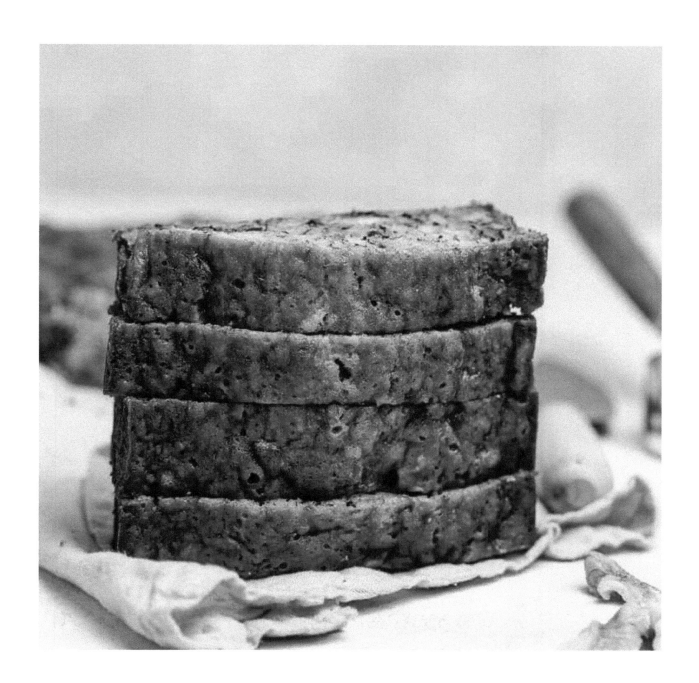

Snacks

MEXICAN WATERMELON SALAD

Watermelon was made for hot summers. It's perfect for picnics and snatched moments in the shade.

MAKES 6 SERVING/ TOTAL TIME 10 MINUTE

INGREDIENTS

4 c Watermelon (cubed)

2 c Jicama (cubed)

Juice from 1 lime

1/4 c Cilantro (fresh chopped)

A dash of ancho chili powder (and/or cayenne- optional)

METHOD

STEP 1

Cube both watermelon and jicama and add to a large serving bowl.

Using a hand juicer, squeeze the juice from your lime over the watermelon and jicama.

STEP 2

Sprinkle fruit bowl with fresh chopped cilantro and mix well.

Garnish with a dash of chili powder and/or cayenne if you're feeling like you want a bit of a kick.

Enjoy!

NUTRITION VALUE	80 Cal, 0.4g fat, 0.04g saturated fat, 5g fiber, 11.3g protein, 14g carbs.

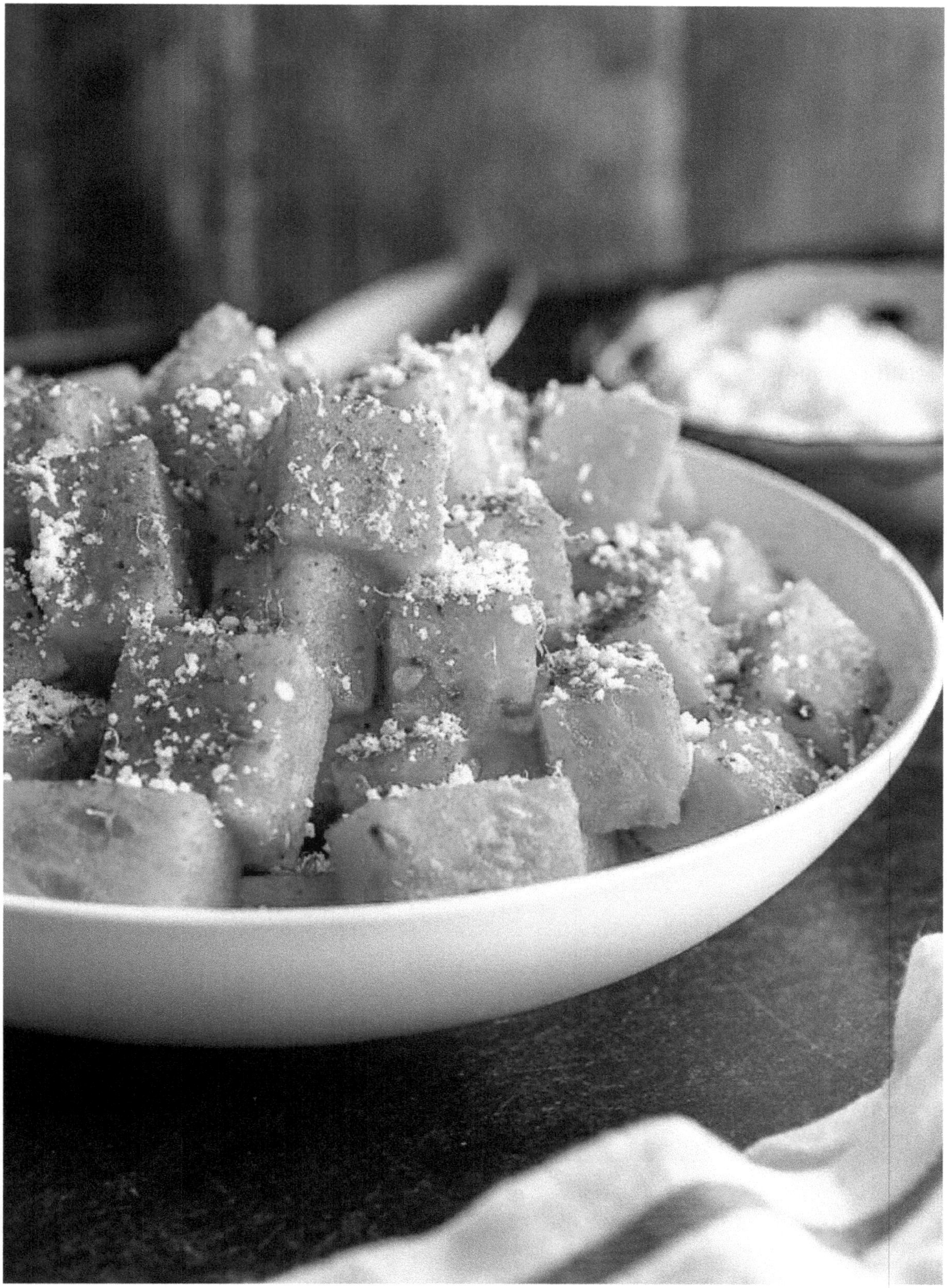

BROILED GRAPEFRUIT PERFECTION

It's spot on for hot summer days when you deserve a treat that tastes, looks, and feels good. Don't go overboard with the fruit but there's no reason you can't enjoy this recipe on a semi-regular basis.

MAKES 2 SERVING/ TOTAL TIME 10 MINUTE

INGREDIENTS

1 Grapefruit (halved)

1 Banana (sliced)

1 tbsp Honey

Cinnamon (to taste)

METHOD

STEP 1

Preheat broiler. Halve grapefruit and slice bananas. Place grapefruit on a baking sheet, and top with the sliced bananas.

STEP 2

Drizzle each piece of grapefruit with 1/2 tbsp honey and sprinkle with cinnamon to taste.

Broil for 5-8 minutes, checking on it occasionally so that it doesn't get burned.

NUTRITION VALUE

1190 KJ Energy, 8.7g fat, 1.9g saturated fat, 13.6g fiber, 11.3g protein, 32.2g carbs.

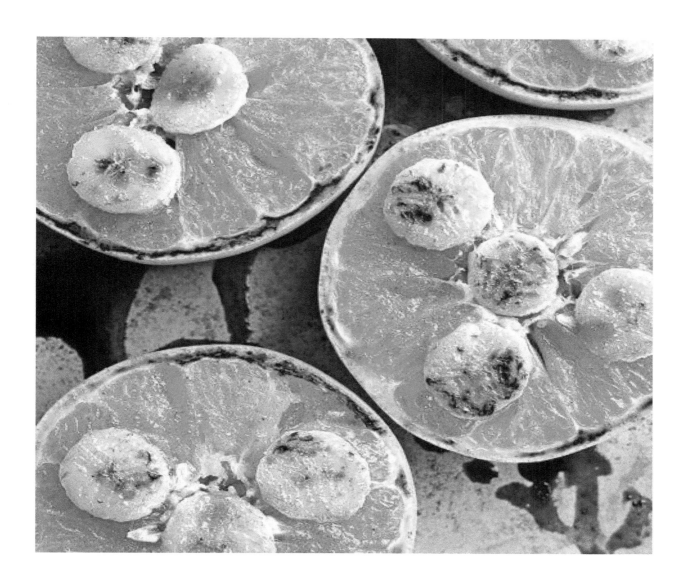

BAKED CABBAGE WEDGES

Try our Baked Cabbage Wedges, either as a snack to keep you going throughout the day, or as a side with some other veggies and a big hunk of meat.

MAKES 2 SERVING/ TOTAL TIME 20 MINUTE

INGREDIENTS

1/2 Head cabbage

6 tbsp Bacon grease

Salt (pepper, garlic powder to taste)

Tin foil

METHOD

STEP 1

Preheat oven to 350 degrees.

Cut 1/2 a head of cabbage into 4 small wedges.

Place wedges in the center of a piece of tin foil.

Cover each of the wedges with 1.5 tbsp of bacon grease, salt, pepper, and garlic powder to taste.

Bake for 1 hour.

NUTRITION VALUE	201 Cal, 20g fat, 9g saturated fat, 13.6g fiber, 22g protein, 13g carbs.

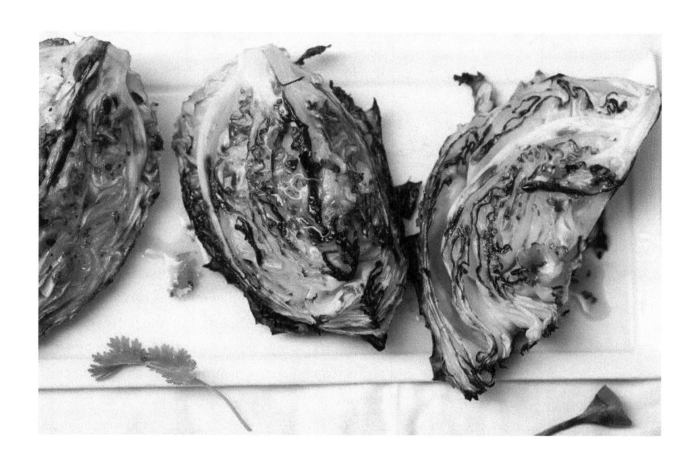

THE ULTIMATE FATTY SLIDER

Recipes That Everyone Love.

MAKES 3 SERVING/ TOTAL TIME 40 MINUTE

INGREDIENTS

1 lb Ground beef

1 tbsp Garlic powder

1 tbsp Onion powder

2 tsp Sea salt

6 strips bacon

2 Avocado (thinly sliced)

1 c Onions (thinly sliced)

3 tbsp Paleo mayo

METHOD

STEP 1

In a large skillet, brown six strips of bacon.
While bacon is cooking, mix ground beef, onion powder, garlic powder, and sea salt together in a large bowl. Form ground beef into six thin patties and set aside. Check on bacon and set aside to cool when finished. Using the bacon fat, sauté onions in the pan. Set aside when complete.

STEP 2

Using the bacon fat, cook burger patties in the pan on a higher heat for about five minutes on each side. Once burgers are complete, top one patty with caramelized onions, two strips of bacon, avocado slices, and 1 tbsp paleo mayo and "sandwich" it with the second patty.

NUTRITION VALUE

495 Cal, 20g fat, 11g saturated fat, 2g fiber, 40g protein, 14g carbs.

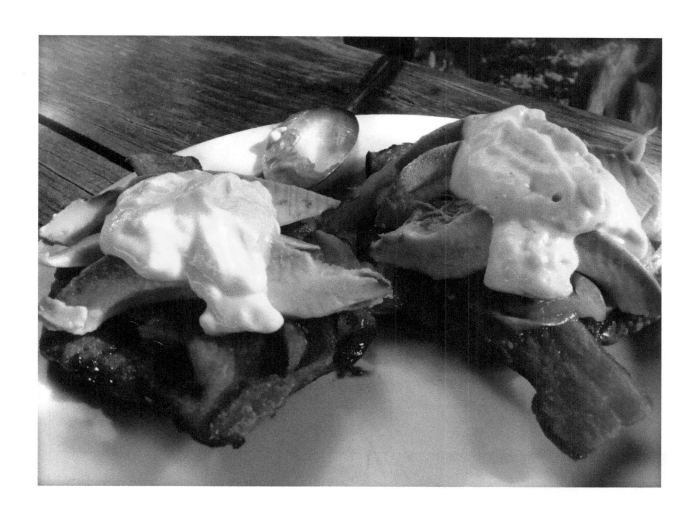

ZESTY VEGGIE DIP

Zesty Veggie Dip packs in plenty of goodness, packs a punch taste-wise, and is super simple to make.

MAKES 1 SERVING/ TOTAL TIME 10 MINUTE

INGREDIENTS

3/4 c Almonds

1/2 c Water

1/3 c Fresh lime juice (about 2 limes)

2 cloves garlic

1/4 c Onion (chopped)

2 tsp Coconut aminos

1 tsp Apple cider vinegar

1/4 tsp Salt

1/4 tsp Smoked paprika

1/4 tsp Dill (dried)

METHOD

STEP 1

Add everything to a blender and puree until a smooth consistency is reached. You might want to rotate between speeds to make sure that all the large chunks are pureed.

STEP 2

Garnish with a sprinkle of paprika and dill.
Serve chilled with veggie sticks. For an extra kick, consider adding cayenne!

NUTRITION VALUE

272 Cal, 20g fat, 2g saturated fat, 6g fiber, 22g protein, 13g carbs.

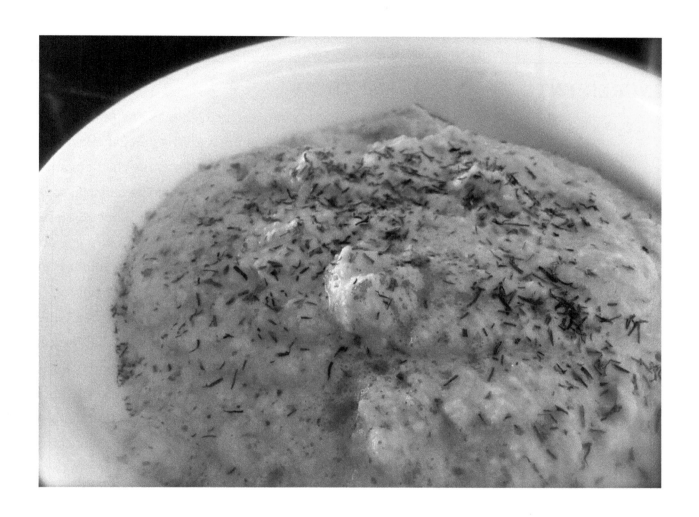

CHICKEN NUGGETS WITH HONEY MUSTARD DIPPING SAUCE

This recipe is ideal both for families whose kids aren't keen on their healthy paleo lifestyle

MAKES 4 SERVING/ TOTAL TIME 30 MINUTE

INGREDIENTS

Nuggets

2 lbs Boneless skinless chicken breasts

1/2 c Vinegar

1 Egg (whisked)

1/4 c Arrowroot powder

1/2 tbsp Paprika

Salt and pepper (to taste)

1 tsp Garlic powder

Cayenne (to taste)

1/2 c Coconut oil (or other preferred cooking fat)

Sauce

1/4 c Yellow mustard

1/4 c Honey

METHOD

Chop chicken into one inch chunks and place into a one gallon Ziplock bag along with the vinegar. Marinate chicken in vinegar for one hour. Take chicken out of the fridge and add the whisked egg to the bag. Massage the chicken and egg mixture in the bag so that all pieces of chicken are covered. Remove excess juice/egg from the bag. In a small dish, mix together dry ingredients and combine well with a fork. Once spices are fully combined, add them to the nuggets in the bag. Seal bag and massage chicken and spices well so that they are fully combined. Combine equal parts of honey and mustard in a small bowl and whisk together using a fork. Heat the coconut oil to high or medium high on the stove in a large pan. Even if you are using your largest pan you might still have to cook the chicken in two batches. It is helpful to have a paper towel lined plate (or two) nearby for the nuggets as they come out of the oil. Cook nuggets for about fifteen minutes allowing seven minutes or so on each side.

Serve as finger food

NUTRITION VALUE	665 Cal, 20g fat, 14g saturated fat, 2g fiber, 52g protein, 8g carbs.

chocolatemoosey.com

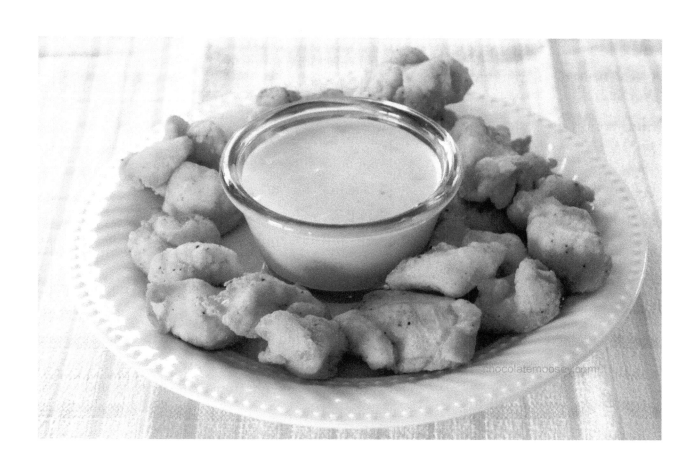

APPLE BROCCOLI SALAD

This salad makes for a filling and fresh snack or side and makes a change from the usual leafy greens plus cucumber and tomatoes job.

MAKES 6 SERVING/ TOTAL TIME 20 MINUTE

INGREDIENTS

Salad

1 Head broccoli (florets, and stem, chopped)

1 Red apple (large, diced)

1 cup Green olives (halved)

1/2 c Red onion (thinly sliced)

1 cup Fresh pineapple

1/4 c Raisins

Vinaigrette

2 cloves garlic

Juice of 2 limes

1/4 c EVOO

2 tbsp Dijon mustard (clean)

1 tbsp White vinegar

2 tbsp Honey

1 tbsp Rosemary

Sea salt and freshly cracked pepper (to taste)

METHOD

STEP 1

In a small blender or food processor, add all the ingredients for the vinaigrette and process until smooth and creamy. Set aside in a small covered jar.

Clean, trim, and roughly chop broccoli. (I used a mandolin slicer to get the stem pieces nice and thin.) Place into a large serving bowl.

STEP 2

Core and dice apple. It's up to you whether you keep the skin or not. Add apple to the broccoli.

Using a mandolin, thinly slice the red onion and add to the broccoli and apple.

Clean, dice, and add pineapple to the salad.

Toss without vinaigrette. Serve the vinaigrette on the side and store separately in the fridge to help preserve the salad.

NUTRITION VALUE

229 Cal, 16g fat, 2g saturated fat, 4g fiber, 21g protein, 12g carbs.

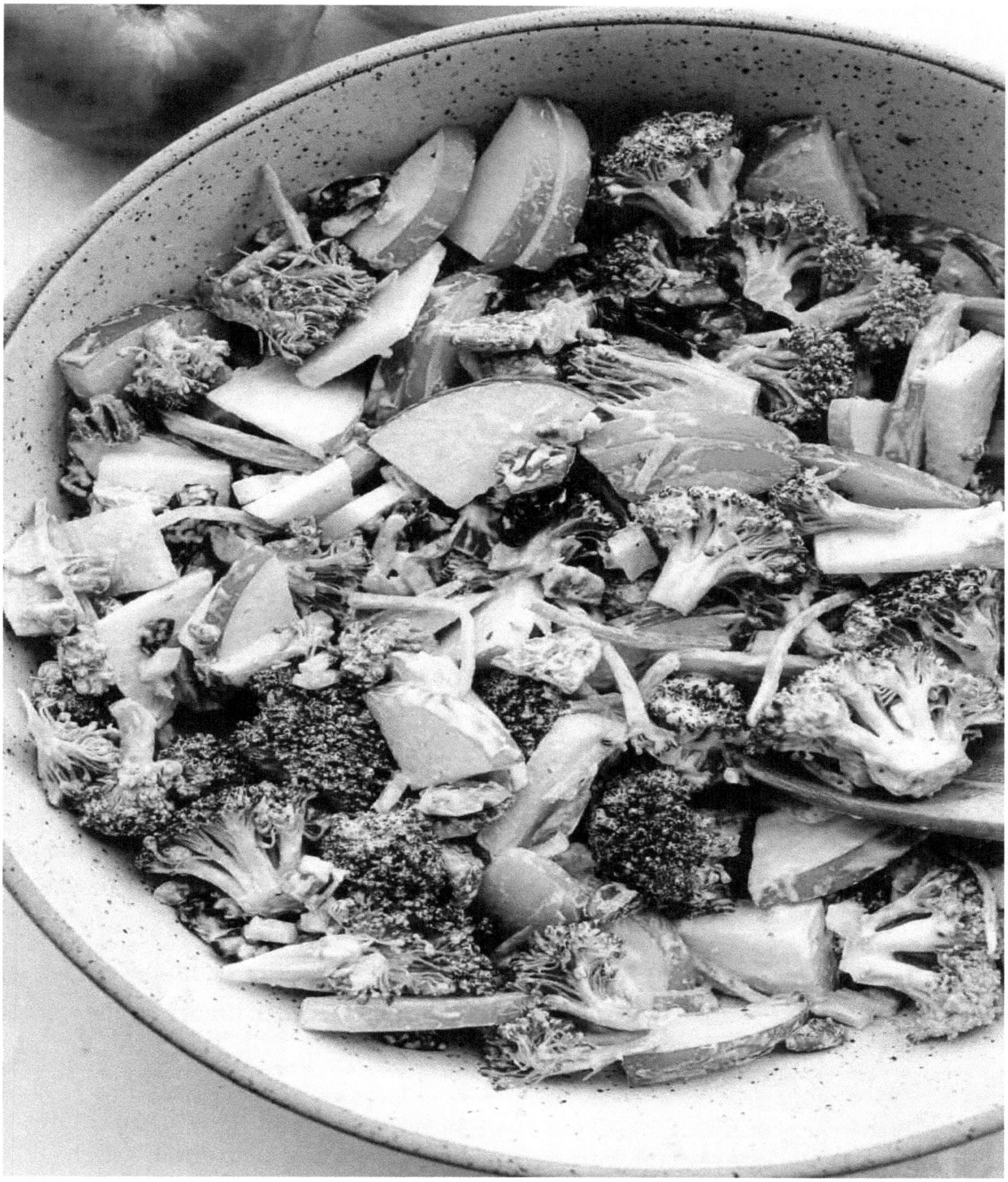

LITERAL EGG ROLL

These egg rolls make great starters, sides, and snacks.

MAKES 1 SERVING/ TOTAL TIME 10 MINUTE

INGREDIENTS

3 Eggs (whisked)

1 tbsp Coconut oil (for frying eggs)

4 sheets Sushi nori/seaweed*

4 tbsp Canned sauerkraut

Salt and pepper (to taste)

Drizzle of sesame oil

METHOD

Melt coconut oil in egg pan.

Pour whisked eggs into frying pan, and add salt, pepper, and seasonings to taste. Cover and cook until eggs reach your desired "done-ness". While eggs are cooking, lay out four sheets of nori, and prepare sauerkraut.

Once eggs are finished, gently and carefully cut them into 2-3 inch strips while they're still in the frying pan. Gently remove a strip of egg using a spatula, and lay it flat about one inch from the top end of the nori sheet. Repeat until all four sheets have a strip of egg.

Use a spoon or fork to evenly place about one tbsp of sauerkraut next to the egg (not on top of the egg).

Lightly drizzle a couple of drops of sesame oil at the top end of the nori sheet nearest the egg. This will make the sheet of nori slightly sticky, so that the roll won't fall apart once you roll it up.

Once rolled, lightly drizzle more sesame oil on the bottom of the nori sheet, and roll everything as tight as the sheet allows. Sesame oil has a strong flavor, so try to use it sparingly. If the sheets don't want to stick together properly, try wetting your fingers with some water from the tap instead of drenching the roll with sesame oil.

NUTRITION VALUE

140 Cal, 15g fat, 14g saturated fat, 13.6g fiber, 21g protein, 8g carbs.

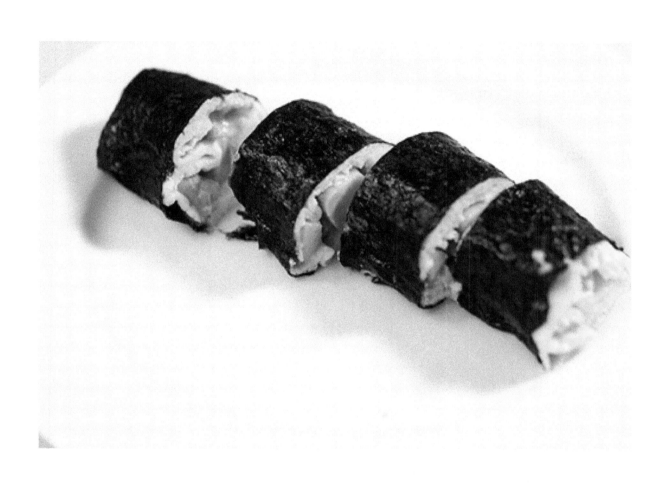

HERB POWER SMOOTHIE

This is a delightful concoction that'll tickle your taste buds.

MAKES 1 SERVING/ TOTAL TIME 10 MINUTE

INGREDIENTS

1 bunch Cilantro

2 cups Kale and spinach (mixed)

1 bunch Fresh parsley

2 Stalks celery

1 Lemon (juiced)

1 1/2 cups Mango (diced)

METHOD

STEP 1

Combine all ingredients in a blender and pulse until smooth.

NUTRITION VALUE	58 Cal, 0.2g fat, 0.1g saturated fat, 2g fiber, 5g protein, 14g carbs.

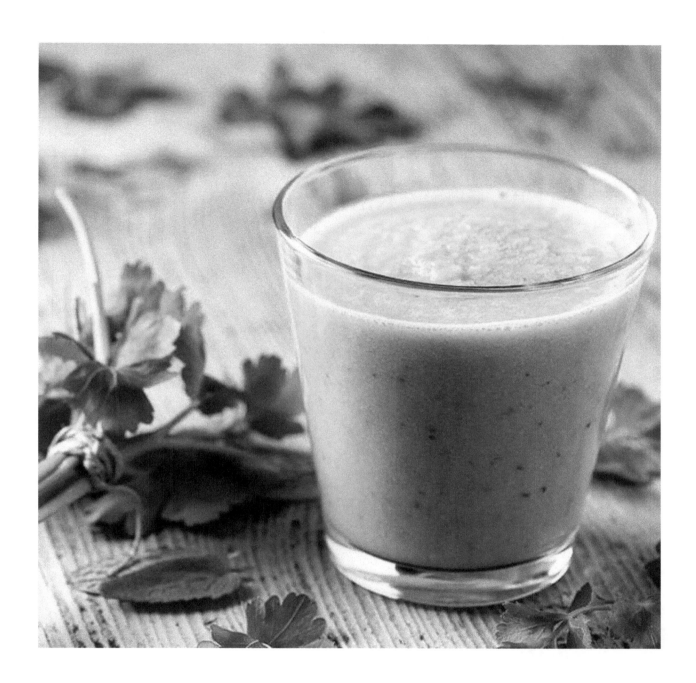

SAVORY GREEN SMOOTHIE

This is a refreshing smoothie for those who like their veggies, but you'll probably want to give it a miss if you're more of a sweet tooth kind of person.

MAKES 1 SERVING/ TOTAL TIME 10 MINUTE

INGREDIENTS

1 cup Spinach

4 Tomatoes

1 cup Water

1 cup Ice

METHOD
STEP 1
Combine all ingredients in a blender and pulse until smooth.

NUTRITION VALUE

14 Cal, 0.2g fat, 0.04g saturated fat, 1g fiber, 9g protein, 2g carbs.

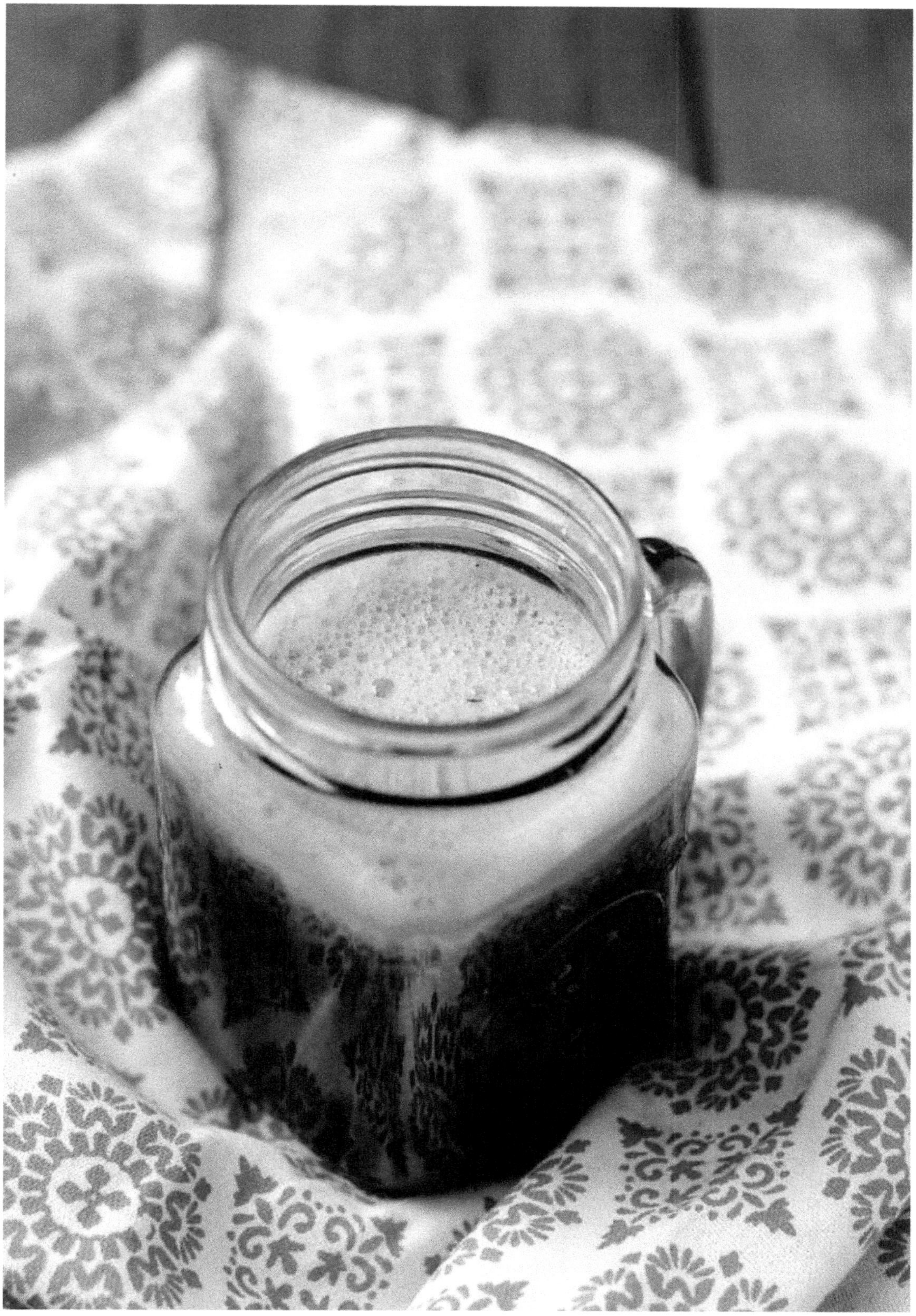

Lightning Source UK Ltd.
Milton Keynes UK
UKHW051004030621
384855UK00002B/318

9 781639 300181